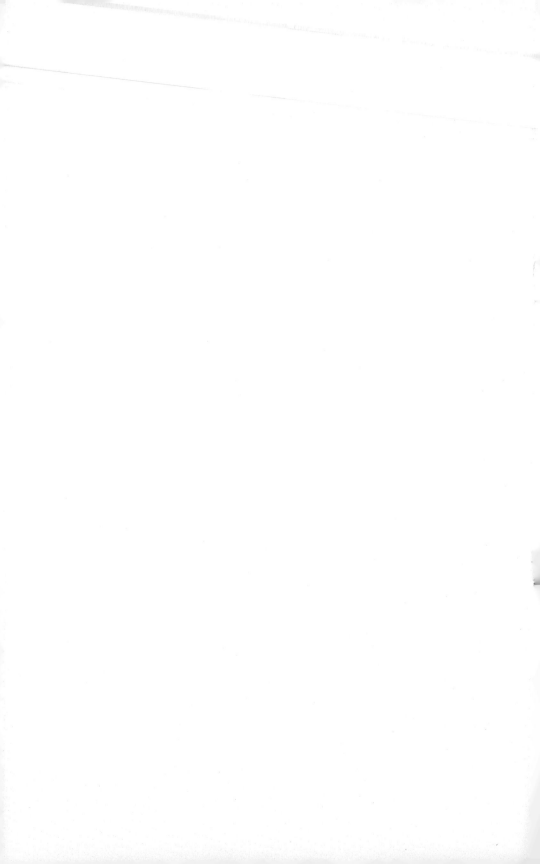

DRY EYE DISEASE

A Practical Guide

DRY EYE DISEASE

A Practical Guide

Editors

Francis S. Mah, MD
Director, Cornea Service
Codirector, Refractive Surgery Service
Scripps Clinic

Michelle K. Rhee, MD
Associate Clinical Professor, Ophthalmology
Cornea, Cataract, and Refractive Surgery
Icahn School of Medicine at Mount Sinai, New York
Medical Director, The Eye-Bank for Sight Restoration, New York
President, CLAO, The Eye and Contact Lens Association

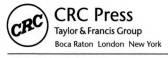

CRC Press
Taylor & Francis Group
Boca Raton London New York

CRC Press is an imprint of the
Taylor & Francis Group, an **informa** business

First published 2019 by SLACK Incorporated

Published 2024 by CRC Press
2385 NW Executive Center Drive, Suite 320, Boca Raton FL 33431

and by CRC Press
4 Park Square, Milton Park, Abingdon, Oxon, OX14 4RN

CRC Press is an imprint of Taylor & Francis Group, LLC

Cover Artist: Justin Dalton

Library of Congress Cataloging-in-Publication Data

Names: Mah, Francis, author. | Rhee, Michelle K., author.
Title: Dry eye disease : a practical guide / Francis S. Mah, Michelle K. Rhee.
Description: Thorofare : Slack Incorporated, 2019. | Includes bibliographical
references and index.
Identifiers: LCCN 2018058002 | ISBN 9781630913779 (paperback)
Subjects: | MESH: Dry Eye Syndromes
Classification: LCC RE216.D78 | NLM WW 208 | DDC 617.7/1--dc23 LC
record available at https://lccn.loc.gov/2018058002

ISBN: 9781630913779 (pbk)
ISBN: 9781003523918 (ebk)

DOI: 10.1201/9781003523918

DEDICATION

To our patients, whose confidence in their doctors motivates the ophthalmic community to continually seek improvements in dry eye care.

To our physician-fathers, Chonggi L. Mah, MD (diagnostic radiology) and Jai Jeen Rhee, MD (cardiology), whose examples have guided and inspired our careers in the humanity and science of medicine.

CONTENTS

ABOUT THE EDITORS

Francis S. Mah, MD has practiced ophthalmology since 2000 with an emphasis in corneal, laser, and cataract surgery.

After undergraduate studies at Cornell University and Dartmouth College, he attended the Medical College of Ohio, graduating at the top of his class. After a residency which included a year as chief resident at the University of Pittsburgh Medical Center, he earned a fellowship in cornea, external disease, and refractive surgery and went on to participate in the clinical research training program. Throughout his academic career, Dr. Mah received numerous awards, such as the Pharmacia and Upjohn Outstanding Resident Award and the American Academy of Ophthalmology Senior Achievement Award.

Upon completion of his training at the University of Pittsburgh Medical Center, Dr. Mah joined the school's faculty, serving as director of the Clinical Vision Research Center and the Charles T. Campbell Ophthalmic Microbiology Laboratory, codirector of the Cornea, External Disease and Refractive Surgery Service, and director of the Cornea and Refractive Surgery Fellowship. Dr. Mah also served as medical director of the Center for Organ Recovery & Education Eye Bank and as team ophthalmologist for the National Football League Pittsburgh Steelers.

Dr. Mah is the author of numerous peer-reviewed articles ranging from dry eye to LASIK surgery to infectious diseases of the external eye. He has published numerous abstracts and delivered a wide range of presentations on 6 continents. Dr. Mah serves in several leadership positions, including chair of the Cornea Clinical Committee, and as a member of the US Food and Drug Administration Committee for American Society of Cataract and Refractive Surgery, and as cochair of the Cornea Preferred Practice Patterns for the American Academy of Ophthalmology. He also completed a 5-year term as the Executive Vice President of Ocular Microbiology and Immunology Group.

Currently, Dr. Mah is the director of the Cornea and External Disease Service, and codirector of the Refractive Surgery Service at Scripps Clinic in La Jolla, California.

Michelle K. Rhee, MD is a cornea and cataract surgeon, with special interests in dry eye, eye banking, and contact lens safety. She is an associate clinical professor of ophthalmology at the Icahn School of Medicine at Mount Sinai, the medical director of the Eye-Bank for Sight Restoration in New York, and the president of the Eye and Contact Lens Association (CLAO). Following studies in piano, cello, and music composition at the Juilliard School, Dr. Rhee graduated *summa cum laude* from Princeton University. She was selected for the early admission humanities and medicine program at the Icahn School of Medicine at Mount Sinai in New York. Dr. Rhee completed her residency at the University of Pittsburgh Medical Center, followed by cornea fellowship at the New York Eye and Ear Infirmary. She also completed training at the

State University of New York Downstate Medical Center in medical acupuncture for physicians.

Dr. Rhee serves on the American Academy of Ophthalmology Ophthalmic News and Education Network, the Preferred Practice Pattern Cornea Panel, and was selected for the 2017 American Academy of Ophthalmology Leadership Development Program. She also chairs the scientific program committee of the Eye Bank Association of America. She has a secondary appointment in the department of medical education at the Icahn School of Medicine, where she directed an ophthalmology elective for medical students. In addition to authoring articles, Dr. Rhee has lectured nationally and internationally on contact lens safety, eye banking, and cataract and refractive surgery.

CONTRIBUTING AUTHORS

Guillermo Amescua, MD (Chapter 9)
Associate Professor of Clinical Ophthalmology
Medical Director of the Ocular Surface Program
Department of Ophthalmology
Bascom Palmer Eye Institute
University of Miami
Miller School of Medicine
Miami, Florida

Alex Barsam, MD (Chapter 10)
Ophthalmology Residency
Department of Ophthalmology
St. Louis University Eye Institute
St. Louis University School of Medicine
St. Louis, Missouri

Ashley R. Brissette, MD, MSc, FRCSC (Chapter 15)
Assistant Professor of Ophthalmology
Department of Ophthalmology
Weill Cornell Medicine
New York, New York

Frank X. Cao, MD (Chapter 12)
Ophthalmologist
Missouri Eye Institute
Joplin, Missouri

Lorenzo J. Cervantes, MD (Chapter 2)
Ophthalmologist
Cornea, External Disease, and Refractive Surgery
Connecticut Eye Specialists
Shelton, Connecticut

Audrey A. Chan, MD, FRCSC (Chapter 8)
Assistant Clinical Professor
Department of Ophthalmology
University of Alberta
Edmonton, Alberta, Canada

Deepinder K. Dhaliwal, MD, LAc (Chapter 19)
Professor of Ophthalmology
Director, Cornea and Refractive Surgery Services
Medical Director, Laser Vision Center
Director and Founder, Center for Integrative Eye Care
Associate Medical Director, Charles T. Campbell Ocular Microbiology Laboratory
University of Pittsburgh Medical Center
Pittsburgh, Pennsylvania
Immediate Past President, CLAO, The Eye and Contact Lens Association

Katherine Duncan, MD (Chapter 5)
Oculoplastic Surgeon
MD EyeCare
Greater Baltimore Medical Center
Towson, Maryland

Marjan Farid, MD (Chapter 1)
Associate Clinical Professor
Gavin Herbert Eye Institute
University of California, Irvine
Irvine, California

Anat Galor, MD, MSPH (Chapter 3)
Associate Professor of Ophthalmology
Bascom Palmer Eye Institute
Department of Ophthalmology
University of Miami
Miami Veterans Administration Medical Center
Miami, Florida

Morgan R. Godin, MD (Chapter 18)
Ophthalmologist
Department of Ophthalmology
Cornea and Refractive Surgery Division
Duke University Eye Center
Durham, North Carolina

Preeya K. Gupta, MD (Chapters 7 & 18)
Associate Professor of Ophthalmology
Duke University School of Medicine
Cornea and External Disease Division
Duke University Eye Center
Durham, North Carolina

Albert S. Hazan, MD (Chapter 11)
Associate Adjunct Surgeon
Department of Ophthalmology
New York Eye and Ear Infirmary of Mount Sinai
New York, New York

Kourtney Houser, MD (Chapter 14)
Assistant Professor of Ophthalmology
University of Tennessee Health Science Center
Memphis, Tennessee

Deborah S. Jacobs, MD (Chapter 16)
Associate Professor of Ophthalmology
Department of Ophthalmology
Massachusetts Eye and Ear
Associate Professor of Ophthalmology
Harvard Medical School
Boston, Massachusetts

Emily J. Jacobs, MD (Chapter 6)
Ophthalmologist
Department of Ophthalmology
New York Eye and Ear Infirmary of Mount Sinai
New York, New York

Bennie H. Jeng, MD (Chapter 17)
Professor and Chair
Department of Ophthalmology and Visual Sciences
University of Maryland School of Medicine
Baltimore, Maryland

Stephen C. Kaufman, MD, PhD (Chapter 12)
Professor of Ophthalmology
Medical College of Wisconsin Eye Institute
Milwaukee, Wisconsin

Michelle J. Kim, MD (Chapter 7)
Clinical Associate
Duke University School of Medicine
Cornea and External Disease Division
Duke University Eye Center
Durham, North Carolina

Terry Kim, MD (Chapter 18)
Professor of Ophthalmology
Duke University School of Medicine
Chief, Cornea and External Disease Division
Director, Refractive Surgery Service
Duke University Eye Center
Durham, North Carolina

Elyse J. McGlumphy, MD (Chapter 17)
Chief Resident
University of Maryland Medical Center
Baltimore, Maryland

Sotiria Palioura, MD, PhD (Chapter 9)
Voluntary Assistant Professor
Department of Ophthalmology
Bascom Palmer Eye Institute
University of Miami
Miller School of Medicine
Miami, Florida

Victor L. Perez, MD (Chapter 10)
Professor of Ophthalmology
Duke Ophthalmology
Duke University School of Medicine
Durham, North Carolina

Stephen C. Pflugfelder, MD (Chapter 14)
Professor and Director, Ocular Surface Center
James and Margaret Elkins Chair
Department of Ophthalmology
Baylor College of Medicine
Houston, Texas

Nataliya Pokeza, MD (Chapter 12)
Ophthalmologist
Wills Eye Hospital
Cornea Service
Corneal Associates, PC
Philadelphia, Pennsylvania

Allison Rizzuti, MD (Chapter 12)
Clinical Assistant Professor
State University of New York Downstate Medical Center
New York, New York

Kelsey Roelofs, MD (Chapter 8)
Ophthalmologist
Department of Ophthalmology
University of Alberta
Edmonton, Alberta, Canada

Bryan Roth, MD (Chapter 4)
Ophthalmology Residency
Baylor College of Medicine
Houston, Texas

John Sheppard, MD, MMSc (Chapter 15)
President, Virginia Eye Consultants
Professor of Ophthalmology
Eastern Virginia Medical School
Norfolk, Virginia

Patricia B. Sierra, MD (Chapter 13)
Ophthalmologist
Cornea, Cataract and Refractive Surgery
Sacramento Eye Consultants
Sacramento, California

Christopher E. Starr, MD (Chapter 15)
Associate Professor of Ophthalmology
Director, Cornea Fellowship
Director, Refractive Surgery Service
Director, Ophthalmic Education
Weill Cornell Medicine
New York Presbyterian Hospital
New York, New York

Christos Theophanous, MD (Chapter 16)
Ophthalmology Residency
Department of Ophthalmology and Visual Science
University of Chicago
Chicago, Illinois

Danielle Trief, MD, MSc (Chapter 11)
Assistant Professor of Ophthalmology
Edward S. Harkness Eye Institute
Columbia University Medical Center
New York, New York

Felipe A. Valenzuela, MD (Chapter 10)
Clinical Fellow
Department of Ophthalmology
Bascom Palmer Eye Institute
University of Miami
Miller School of Medicine
Miami, Florida

Nandini Venkateswaran, MD (Chapter 3)
Ophthalmology Residency
Bascom Palmer Eye Institute
University of Miami
Miami, Florida

Elizabeth Viriya, MD (Chapter 15)
Clinical Assistant Professor
Department of Ophthalmology
NYU Langone Medical Center
New York, New York

Priscilla Q. Vu, MD, MS (Chapter 1)
Ophthalmology Residency
University of California, Irvine
Irvine, California

Walt Whitley, OD, MBA (Chapter 15)
Director of Optometric Services
Residency Program Supervisor
Virginia Eye Consultants
Norfolk, Virginia

Elizabeth Yeu, MD (Chapter 4)
Assistant Professor of Ophthalmology
Eastern Virginia Medical School
Partner, Virginia Eye Consultants
Medical Director
Cornea, Cataract, Anterior Segment and Refractive Surgery
Virginia Surgery Center
Norfolk, Virginia

Jenny Y. Yu, MD, FACS (Chapter 5)
Assistant Professor
Oculoplastics, Orbital, and Aesthetics Surgery
Department of Ophthalmology and Otolaryngology
University of Pittsburgh Medical Center
Pittsburgh, Pennsylvania

Siwei Zhou, MD (Chapter 19)
Ophthalmology Residency
University of Pittsburgh Medical Center
Pittsburgh, Pennsylvania

PREFACE

Dry Eye Disease: A Practical Guide was written to review, guide, and update physicians with a practical and clinically oriented source for treating the growing population of dry eye patients. From epidemiology and pathogenesis, to disease subgroups, diagnostics, and management, our goal was to provide comprehensive scientific information, while also structuring it as user-friendly for a busy clinical practice. We have highlighted key information as take home points, and clinical scenarios are used to engage the reader to critically think and apply current understanding of dry eye disease to the office and operating room. It is our hope that ophthalmologists and optometrists of all specialties (and at all stages of training and practice) will find this of interest as we also discuss the relationship of dry eye disease to surgical outcomes and contact lens wear. *Dry Eye Disease: A Practical Guide* is SLACK's first book on this topic following the 2007 and 2017 full reports of the International Dry Eye WorkShop (DEWS I and II), which were turning points in the understanding of this complex disease. We also include information on the latest biomarker diagnostics, meibomian gland dysfunction therapeutic technologies, and integrative medicine.

As this book was going to press, the Dry Eye Assessment and Management (DREAM) trial was presented at the American Society of Cataract and Refractive Surgery meeting in Washington DC. After its publication in *The New England Journal of Medicine*[1], we reassessed our text, especially with regard to the use of omega-3 fatty acids. We applaud the researchers' diligence in examining the value of omega-3 fatty acids. While this study certainly enhances our understanding of dry eye disease, it does not obviate the use of all omega-3 fatty acids, which remain an important treatment option for dry eye disease.

We are grateful to our expert and experienced contributing authors for the hard work and generous thoughtfulness put into sharing their knowledge. To reflect a diversity of perspectives, we recruited leaders in the field throughout North America from a variety of practice settings including university-based and private.

Tony Schiavo, Julia Dolinger, and Joseph Lowery, with their exceptional team at SLACK, have shepherded this book to fruition with their exemplary organizational and motivational skills.

Finally, we are thankful to our families for their endless love and support.

—Francis S. Mah, MD
—Michelle K. Rhee, MD

REFERENCE

1. Dry Eye Assessment and Management Study Research Group, Asbell PA, Maguire MG, et al. n-3 fatty acid supplementation for the treatment of dry eye disease. *N Engl J Med*. 2018;3;378(18):1681-1690.

SECTION I

SETTING THE STAGE

CHAPTER 1

Epidemiology
Incidence, Prevalence, and Impact of Disease

Priscilla Q. Vu, MD, MS and Marjan Farid, MD

KEY POINTS

- The prevalence of dry eye disease (DED) ranges from 5% to 34% globally.
- The most consistent risk factors for DED are older age and female sex.
- Severe DED affects patient quality of life in a manner equivalent to patients with angina pectoris, dialysis, and hip fractures.
- One study found the costs of DED management to be approximately $783 per person per year in the United States, amounting to $3.84 million per year.

As our understanding and ability to diagnose dry eye disease (DED) improves, the ophthalmic community is realizing that larger than previously reported proportions of the population are affected by this disease. There are a variety of risk factors associated with DED, and our understanding of which patients are likely to get DED continues to improve. DED can have a significant impact on quality of life, making efficient and effective management crucial. This chapter will explore our current understanding of these topics.

Mah FS, Rhee MK, eds.
Dry Eye Disease: A Practical Guide (pp 3-9).
© 2019 Taylor & Francis Group.

PREVALENCE AND INCIDENCE

The prevalence of DED ranges from 5% to 34% and affects a diverse, global population.[1] Studies describing the incidence of DED are scarce. In the Women's Health Study, one of the largest cross-sectional studies on DED in the United States, the age-adjusted prevalence of DED in women over 50 years old was 7.8% or 3.23 million (N = 39,876).[2] In another large study by the Physician Health Studies, prevalence of DED for men over 50 years old in the United States was 1.68 million (N = 25,444).[3] Differences in prevalence among studies can be attributed to differences in diagnosis, variations in sample populations, variability in disease process, and the subjective nature of symptoms.[1] In 2007, DED was first clearly defined by the International Dry Eye WorkShop as "a multifactorial disease of the tears and ocular surface that results in symptoms of discomfort, visual disturbance, and tear film instability with potential damage to the ocular surface. It is accompanied by increased osmolarity of the tear film and inflammation of the ocular surface."[4] This definition has improved the ability to study DED prevalence; however, studies remain limited by geographic and population differences.

The majority of patients with DED have 1 of 3 subtypes: evaporative dry eye (EDE), aqueous-tear deficient dry eye (ADDE; Sjögren syndrome and non-Sjögren syndrome), and combined EDE and ADDE.[4] A retrospective study of 299 patients found 71% of patients with one of these subtypes.[5] Current studies suggest EDE or a mixed EDE/ADDE form is more common, and that meibomian gland dysfunction is the most common cause of EDE.[5,6]

RISK FACTORS

Although risk factors vary among studies, the most consistent risk factors for DED are older age and female sex.[1-3] Women are almost twice as likely as men to have DED.[2,3] The Women's Health Study found DED to increase with age from 5.7% among women under 50 years old to 9.8% in women over 75 years old.[2] There are also many other risk factors, including hormonal imbalances or fluctuations, systemic diseases, infections, cancer treatments, prior ophthalmic surgery, medication use, nutritional deficiencies, and environmental exposures (Table 1-1).[1]

Additionally, certain work and living environments are associated with DED. In India, tannery workers who have chemical exposures and work in a hot, dusty environment were more likely to have DED.[7] In Korea, urban dwellers and those in areas with low humidity and longer sunshine duration were more likely to have DED.[8] In a Japanese study, up to 60% of computer users were diagnosed with DED.[9] In Ghana, DED symptoms were most likely in patients who lived in windy conditions, low humidity, and air-conditioned rooms.[10] In developed countries, the increased use of computer and device screens may also be a contributing factor to the rise of DED.[1,9]

Of note, DED is also related to a variety of comorbidities. A Taiwanese study found a variety of comorbidities associated with DED, including ischemic heart disease, hyperlipidemia, cardiac arrhythmias, peripheral vascular disease, stroke, migraine, myasthenia

TABLE 1-1

RISK FACTORS FOR DRY EYE DISEASE	
Female Sex	**Ophthalmic Surgery**
Older Age	Refractive surgery
Hormonal	Keratoplasty
Androgen deficiency	**Medication Use**
Ovarian failure	Antihistamines
Hormone replacement therapy	Antidepressants
Systemic Diseases	Beta-blockers
Autoimmune/connective tissue diseases	Diuretics
	Anticholinergics
Sjögren syndrome	Isotretinoin
Rheumatoid arthritis	**Nutritional Deficiency**
Graves' disease	Vitamin A deficiency
Diabetes mellitus	Omega-3 and omega-6 deficiency
Sarcoidosis	**Environmental**
Infections	Low humidity or windy environments
HIV/HTLV-1 infections	
Hepatitis C	Urban settings
Oncology Related	Industrial exposures
Bone marrow transplantation (graft-versus-host disease)	Visual display terminal/computer use
Radiation therapy	Contact lens wear
Chemotherapy	

gravis, rheumatoid arthritis, systemic lupus erythematosus, asthma, pulmonary circulation disorders, diabetes with complications, hypothyroidism, liver disease, peptic ulcer disease, hepatitis B, deficiency anemia, depression, psychoses, and solid tumors without metastases.[11] A British study found DED to be associated with age, asthma, eczema, allergies, cataract surgery, rheumatoid arthritis, osteoarthritis, migraine, stroke, depression, pelvic pain, irritable bowel syndrome, and chronic widespread pain syndrome.[12] Our understanding of these comorbidities and their relationship to DED remains limited.

TABLE 1-2

IMPACT OF DRY EYE DISEASE	
Difficulty With Activities of Daily Living	**Quality of Life Decrease**
Reading	Chronic debilitating symptoms
Driving	Anxiety and depression
Loss in Work Productivity	**Management Costs**

IMPACT OF DISEASE

DED is a chronic, lifelong disease and many patients will report progressively worsening ocular surface symptoms, vision-related symptoms, and social impact once diagnosed.[13] Ocular surface symptoms include frequency and severity of symptoms, such as eye dryness and irritation, dissatisfaction with treatment, and overall severity of condition.[13] Vision-related symptoms include perceived vision quality and interference with activities of daily living.[13] Social impact refers to the ability to socialize and overall mood.[13] Patients with DED will have increased difficulty with activities of daily living, decreased quality of life, and decreased work productivity. Furthermore, patients with DED are more likely to have depression and anxiety disorders. DED can thus present a huge cost to society and productivity, making efficient management crucial (Table 1-2).

Activities of Daily Living and Work Productivity

Studies have found patients to have significant reductions in functional reading on the computer and driving.[14,15] DED is associated with reduced reading speed[16] and reduced driving reaction time.[17] A cross-sectional web-based survey found DED severity is associated with work productivity loss and impairment of daily activities (N = 9034).[18] In the United States, a prospective, cross-sectional study of 158 DED patients naïve to prescription medications found loss in 0.36% work time (approximately 5 minutes over 7 days) and approximately 30% performance impairment, work place productivity, and non–job-related activities.[19] Although actual absent days from work are marginal, the estimated loss in work productivity is profound.

Quality of Life and Mood Disorders

Utility assessments are formal methods to understanding the relative impact of a given health status or disease on patient lives, and have been applied to DED patients.[20,21] These studies have found severe DED to affect patient quality of life in a manner equivalent to patients with angina pectoris, dialysis, and hip fractures.[20,21] In a variety of questionnaires, patients with DED have consistently expressed a reduction in quality of life compared to their healthy counterparts.[15,20-24] Fatigue and pain scores as well as mental health and social functioning scores were reduced in patients with DED.[1] Subjective patient questionnaires validate that increased objective disease severity is correlated with perceived reduction in quality of life.[25] Another study found that patients had DED symptoms interfering with leisure activities 123 days per year.[26]

DED is also associated with anxiety and depression disorders.[27-30] Meta-analysis of 22 studies of approximately 2.9 million patients found prevalence of depression and anxiety to be greater in DED than in controls, and greatest in primary Sjögren syndrome patients.[31]

Costs

One study found the costs of DED management to be approximately $783 per person per year in the United States, amounting to $3.84 million per year.[32] In a study of 6 European countries, 1000 DED patients managed by ophthalmologists ranged in costs from $0.27 million in France to $1.10 million in the United Kingdom.[33] These costs include clinic visits, diagnostic tests, and treatments.[33] Prescription costs ranged from $22 per person per year in France to $535 per person per year in the United Kingdom.[33] In Asia, annual per person drug cost was $323 ± 219 US dollars, clinical cost was $165 ± 101 US dollars, and total direct cost was $530 ± 384.[34] In Singapore, total annual expenditure in 2008 and 2009 was more than $1.5 million and about $22 to $24 per person.[35] These costs are expected to increase with population growth.

Indirect annual costs in the United States from decreased work productivity are estimated to be $11,302 per person, with an overall cost burden of $55.4 billion.[32] Missed workdays due to DED symptoms are 8.2 days for mild symptoms and up to 14.2 days per year for severe DED.[32] Work productivity loss was 91 days for mild DED and up to 128.2 days for severe DED.[32] In Japan, annual cost per person by indirect cost analysis was around $741 per person from loss in work productivity.[36] Another study found that patients with DED missed 5 days of work over a year due to symptoms, and had symptoms at work 208 days over a year.[26] In Japan, work productivity decreased about $6160 per employee when measured by total production and $1178 per employee when calculated by wage.[37]

Also, based on recent trends, costs are expected to increase in the future and be greater for women than men.[38,39] Women were more likely to pursue treatments, have increased costs, and also report greater dissatisfaction with treatments than men.[38] In one study, mean medication expenditure of topical cyclosporine A and sulfacetamide-prednisolone for DED increased from 2001 to 2006 from $55 to $299, with females spending more than males ($244 vs $122).[39]

Summary

DED affects up to one-third of the population, but true prevalence values remain elusive given variability in study populations and diagnosis of DED. With continued advances in diagnostic and treatment options and further studies into the pathophysiology of disease, we will be able to identify these patients more readily in our practices. The physician's role in managing DED expands through all specialties of eye care, and the larger impact on quality of life and productivity can be greatly influenced by continued progress in DED management.

References

1. The epidemiology of dry eye disease: report of the Epidemiology Subcommittee of the International Dry Eye WorkShop (2007). *Ocul Surf.* 2007;5(2):93-107.
2. Schaumberg DA, Sullivan DA, Buring JE, Dana MR. Prevalence of dry eye syndrome among US women. *Am J Ophthalmol.* 2003;136(2):318-326.
3. Schaumberg DA, Dana R, Buring JE, Sullivan DA. Prevalence of dry eye disease among US men: estimates from the Physicians' Health Studies. *Arch Ophthalmol.* 2009;127(6):763-768.
4. The definition and classification of dry eye disease: report of the Definition and Classification Subcommittee of the International Dry Eye WorkShop (2007). *Ocul Surf.* 2007;5(2):75-92.
5. Lemp MA, Crews LA, Bron AJ, Foulks GN, Sullivan BD. Distribution of aqueous-deficient and evaporative dry eye in a clinic-based patient cohort: a retrospective study. *Cornea.* 2012;31(5):472-478.
6. Bron AJ, Tomlinson A, Foulks GN, et al. Rethinking dry eye disease: a perspective on clinical implications. *Ocul Surf.* 2014;12(2 Suppl):S1-S31.
7. Gupta RC, Ranjan R, Kushwaha RN, Khan P, Mohan S. A questionnaire-based survey of dry eye disease among leather tannery workers in Kanpur, India: a case-control study. *Cutan Ocul Toxicol.* 2014;33(4):265-269.
8. Um SB, Kim NH, Lee HK, Song JS, Kim HC. Spatial epidemiology of dry eye disease: findings from South Korea. *Int J Health Geogr.* 2014;13:31.
9. Kawashima M, Yamatsuji M, Yokoi N, et al. Screening of dry eye disease in visual display terminal workers during occupational health examinations: the Moriguchi study. *J Occup Health.* 2015;57(3):253-258.
10. Asiedu K, Kyei S, Boampong F, Ocansey S. Symptomatic dry eye and its associated factors: a study of university undergraduate students in Ghana. *Eye Contact Lens.* 2017;43(4):262-266.
11. Wang TJ, Wang IJ, Hu CC, Lin HC. Comorbidities of dry eye disease: a nationwide population-based study. *Acta Ophthalmol.* 2012;90(7):663-668.
12. Vehof J, Kozareva D, Hysi PG, Hammond CJ. Prevalence and risk factors of dry eye disease in a British female cohort. *Br J Ophthalmol.* 2014;98(12):1712-1717.
13. Lienert JP, Tarko L, Uchino M, Christen WG, Schaumberg DA. Long-term natural history of dry eye disease from the patient's perspective. *Ophthalmology.* 2016;123(2):425-433.
14. Liu Z, Pflugfelder SC. Corneal surface regularity and the effect of artificial tears in aqueous tear deficiency. *Ophthalmology.* 1999;106(5):939-943.
15. Miljanovic B, Dana R, Sullivan DA, Schaumberg DA. Impact of dry eye syndrome on vision-related quality of life. *Am J Ophthalmol.* 2007;143(3):409-415.
16. Ridder WH 3rd, Zhang Y, Huang JF. Evaluation of reading speed and contrast sensitivity in dry eye disease. *Optom Vis Sci.* 2013;90(1):37-44.
17. Deschamps N, Ricaud X, Rabut G, Labbe A, Baudouin C, Denoyer A. The impact of dry eye disease on visual performance while driving. *Am J Ophthalmol.* 2013;156(1):184-189.e183.
18. Patel VD, Watanabe JH, Strauss JA, Dubey AT. Work productivity loss in patients with dry eye disease: an online survey. *Curr Med Res Opin.* 2011;27(5):1041-1048.

19. Nichols KK, Bacharach J, Holland E, et al. Impact of dry eye disease on work productivity, and patients' satisfaction with over-the-counter dry eye treatments. *Invest Ophthalmol Vis Sci.* 2016;57(7):2975-2982.

20. Schiffman RM, Walt JG, Jacobsen G, Doyle JJ, Lebovics G, Sumner W. Utility assessment among patients with dry eye disease. *Ophthalmology.* 2003;110(7):1412-1419.

21. Buchholz P, Steeds CS, Stern LS, et al. Utility assessment to measure the impact of dry eye disease. *Ocul Surf.* 2006;4(3):155-161.

22. Friedman NJ. Impact of dry eye disease and treatment on quality of life. *Curr Opin Ophthalmol.* 2010;21(4):310-316.

23. Rajagopalan K, Abetz L, Mertzanis P, et al. Comparing the discriminative validity of two generic and one disease-specific health-related quality of life measures in a sample of patients with dry eye. *Value Health.* 2005;8(2):168-174.

24. Li M, Gong L, Chapin WJ, Zhu M. Assessment of vision-related quality of life in dry eye patients. *Invest Ophthalmol Vis Sci.* 2012;53(9):5722-5727.

25. Garcia-Catalan MR, Jerez-Olivera E, Benitez-Del-Castillo-Sanchez JM. [Dry eye and quality of life]. *Arch Soc Esp Oftalmol.* 2009;84(9):451-458.

26. Hirsch JD. Considerations in the pharmacoeconomics of dry eye. *Manag Care.* 2003;12(12 Suppl):S33-S38.

27. Li M, Gong L, Sun X, Chapin WJ. Anxiety and depression in patients with dry eye syndrome. *Curr Eye Res.* 2011;36(1):1-7.

28. Labbe A, Wang YX, Jie Y, Baudouin C, Jonas JB, Xu L. Dry eye disease, dry eye symptoms and depression: the Beijing Eye Study. *Br J Ophthalmol.* 2013;97(11):1399-1403.

29. Paulsen AJ, Cruickshanks KJ, Fischer ME, et al. Dry eye in the beaver dam offspring study: prevalence, risk factors, and health-related quality of life. *Am J Ophthalmol.* 2014;157(4):799-806.

30. Na KS, Han K, Park YG, Na C, Joo CK. Depression, stress, quality of life, and dry eye disease in Korean women: A population-based study. *Cornea.* 2015;34(7):733-738.

31. Wan KH, Chen LJ, Young AL. Depression and anxiety in dry eye disease: a systematic review and meta-analysis. *Eye (Lond).* 2016;30(12):1558-1567.

32. Yu J, Asche CV, Fairchild CJ. The economic burden of dry eye disease in the United States: a decision tree analysis. *Cornea.* 2011;30(4):379-387.

33. Clegg JP, Guest JF, Lehman A, Smith AF. The annual cost of dry eye syndrome in France, Germany, Italy, Spain, Sweden and the United Kingdom among patients managed by ophthalmologists. *Ophthalmic Epidemiol.* 2006;13(4):263-274.

34. Mizuno Y, Yamada M, Shigeyasu C. Annual direct cost of dry eye in Japan. *Clin Ophthalmol.* 2012;6:755-760.

35. Waduthantri S, Yong SS, Tan CH, et al. Cost of dry eye treatment in an Asian clinic setting. *PloS One.* 2012;7(6):e37711.

36. Yamada M, Mizuno Y, Shigeyasu C. Impact of dry eye on work productivity. *Clinicoecon Outcomes Res.* 2012;4:307-312.

37. Uchino M, Yokoi N, Uchino Y, et al. Prevalence of dry eye disease and its risk factors in visual display terminal users: the Osaka study. *Am J Ophthalmol.* 2013;156(4):759-766.

38. Schaumberg DA, Uchino M, Christen WG, Semba RD, Buring JE, Li JZ. Patient reported differences in dry eye disease between men and women: impact, management, and patient satisfaction. *PloS One.* 2013;8(9):e76121.

39. Galor A, Zheng DD, Arheart KL, et al. Dry eye medication use and expenditures: data from the medical expenditure panel survey 2001 to 2006. *Cornea.* 2012;31(12):1403-1407.

CHAPTER 2

Pathogenesis and Classification

Lorenzo J. Cervantes, MD

KEY POINTS

- The definition of dry eye disease (DED) continues to evolve since its description in 1930. Most recently, tear film homeostasis is at the core of the definition.
- Inflammation and hyperosmolarity are integral parts of the pathophysiology of DED, as both result from and contribute to the perpetuation of the "vicious cycle."
- There are 4 main subtypes of DED: aqueous deficiency, meibomian gland dysfunction, mucin deficiency, and exposure related.
- Co-conspirators masquerade as or exacerbate DED. These include medicamentosa, ocular allergy, conjunctivochalasis, contact lens wear.
- Symptoms of DED include ocular discomfort, dryness, burning/stinging, foreign body sensation, photophobia, and blurred/fluctuating vision.

Duke-Elder coined the term *keratitis sicca* in 1930 to describe a "condition associated with a deficiency of lacrimal secretion" characterized by "punctiform opacities, sometimes with filaments, and usually accompanied by a chronic conjunctivitis characterized by a small amount of viscous secretion."[1] Based on previous case reports, he surmised

Mah FS, Rhee MK, eds.
Dry Eye Disease: A Practical Guide (pp 11-24).
© 2019 Taylor & Francis Group.

that this condition occurred congenitally,[2] after trauma or surgery,[3,4] or in postmenopausal women.[5]

Since that time, the definition of dry eye disease (DED) has evolved and the associations to it are almost too numerous to count. Patients with symptoms consistent with DED might present in a straightforward manner (eg, "My eyes only feel dry when I play video games for a long time"). For others, it can be more complicated (eg, "My eyes have always been dry since my cataract and LASIK surgeries, I have a new stye, and my rheumatologist says that my rheumatoid arthritis has been acting up"). Because of the implications DED can have on activities of daily living and mental health,[6,7] because treatment for various forms of DED are becoming more expensive,[8,9] and because physicians are also increasingly frustrated in treating more advanced cases of DED,[10] it behooves us to understand DED as anything but simple.

In this chapter, we will examine the pathogenesis of DED, first by defining the functional units necessary to maintain a healthy ocular surface, then by understanding the implications their dysfunction has on the ocular surface. This puts into motion a vicious cycle that, once entered, has the effect of perpetuating a worsening disease state that becomes more difficult to treat over time. We will also define the latest classifications of the various forms of DED to better recognize and address them.

How Do We Define Dry Eye?

By its simple moniker, "dry eye disease" does very little to describe its complex nature. Its definition has evolved to reflect this. In 1995, the National Eye Institute/Industry Workshop on Clinical Trials in Dry Eyes called it "a disorder of the tear film due to tear deficiency or excessive tear evaporation which causes damage to the interpalpebral ocular surface and is associated with symptoms of ocular discomfort."[11] In 2007, the International Dry Eye WorkShop defined dry eye as "a multifactorial disease of the tears and ocular surface that results in symptoms of discomfort, visual disturbance, and tear film instability with potential damage to the ocular surface; it is accompanied by increased osmolarity of the tear film and inflammation of the ocular surface."[12] The updated Preferred Practice Pattern guidelines from the American Academy of Ophthalmology pertaining to dry eye and blepharitis[13] state that "dry eye syndrome refers to a group of disorders of the tear film that are due to reduced tear production or excessive tear evaporation, associated with ocular discomfort and/or visual symptoms and possible disease of the ocular surface." In addition to keratitis or keratoconjunctivitis sicca, DED has also been called *dysfunctional tear syndrome* (DTS), a term coined in 2006 by the Dysfunctional Tear Syndrome Study Group.[14] "Keratoconjunctivitis sicca," "dry eye disease," and "dysfunctional tear syndrome" have been used in lieu of each other.

In 2017, the definition evolved to emphasize the departure from normal tear film as an essential attribute to the pathophysiology of DED. The Cornea, External Disease, and Refractive Society convened a specialty panel[15] calling DTS "a disorder of the tear film in quality and/or quantity, which is caused by a range of etiologies and involves abnormalities in one or more components of the tear film, resulting in a constellation

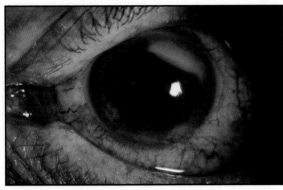

Figure 2-1. A mixed picture. Although this patient presented acutely with corneal marginal infiltrates, the underlying pathology should not be ignored. Her meibomian glands are congested and inflamed, and her lower eyelid shows severe laxity. Failure to address all these issues can lead to recurrent episodes and an overall worsening of symptoms.

of signs and symptoms affecting the ocular surface. Any alteration in the quantity and/or quality of the tear film can result in DTS, a chronic condition with multiple subtypes that include DED and associated tear film disorders." The International Dry Eye WorkShop defined dry eye as "a multifactorial disease of the ocular surface characterized by a loss of homeostasis of the tear film, and accompanied by ocular symptoms, in which tear film instability and hyperosmolarity, ocular surface inflammation and damage, and neurosensory abnormalities play etiological roles."[16]

PATHOGENESIS—HOW DOES IT HAPPEN?

In its normal state, the lacrimal and accessory glands, eyelids, meibomian glands, conjunctiva, cornea, and tear film all contribute to the health and stability of the ocular surface. Dysfunction of any of these components, in addition to desiccating stress, can lead to a compromise in the tear film, hyperosmolarity, increased friction, and chronic mechanical irritation, affecting the various components of the ocular surface (Figure 2-1). A perpetuating vicious cycle ensues, with inflammation and hyperosmolarity playing an integral role. Symptoms of DED result from stimulation and irritation of the trigeminal sensory neurons and include ocular discomfort, dryness, burning, foreign body sensation, photophobia, and blurred/fluctuating vision.[15,16]

Lacrimal Gland

The main lacrimal gland consists of a larger orbital lobe and a smaller palpebral lobe that produces the bulk of serous secretions that become the aqueous component of the tear film. Accessory lacrimal glands of Krause and Wolfring constitute about 10% of the total lacrimal tissue mass.[17] Both main and accessory glands are innervated by parasympathetic and sympathetic nervous system pathways whereby a neural reflex arc originating from the ocular surface[18-21] and the nasal mucosa[22] stimulate secretion. Immune cells, including B and T cells, dendritic cells, macrophages, monocytes, and mast cells, significantly occupy the gland's interstitial space.[23] Damage to the gland (eg, from radiation exposure or autoimmune processes) causes immune cell infiltration and glandular cell loss.[24]

Eyelids

The eyelids serve to protect the ocular surface by cleaning and lubricating the eyes, providing a physical barrier from desiccation and external sources of injury. The skin provides the outermost barrier for protection. The eyelashes prevent debris from reaching the ocular surface. The underlying orbicularis oculi aid in eyelid closure, contribute to the lacrimal pump,[16] and hold the lacrimal punctum against the sclera for proper drainage of tears.[25] The tarsal plates provide structural stability of the eyelids and contain the meibomian glands. A lesion of the facial nerve can cause eyelid paralysis, such as in Bell's palsy. Degeneration and laxity of the tarsal plates can lead to eyelid malposition (ectropion/entropion). A normal spontaneous blink occurs between 15 and 20 times per minute.[26] The blink rate increases in DED and decreases with neurotrophic corneas or with activities such as driving, reading, watching television, operating monitor-based and hand-held video games, and performing surgery,[27-31] potentiating desiccating stress.

Tear Film

With the eyes open, tears are distributed among 3 compartments—within the fornices, the tear menisci, and the tear film.[16] The tear film is responsible for lubrication, protection from disease, nutrition of the cornea, and providing a refractive interface.[32] Tears consists of 3 main components—aqueous, mucin, and lipid. The aqueous component contains proteins and electrolytes and is largely a product of the lacrimal gland. Low tear meniscus volume is correlated with low total tear fluid volume and lacrimal secretory rate.[33,34] The mucinous component functions to promote adherence of the tear film to the ocular surface and is made by the conjunctival goblet cells and conjunctival and corneal epithelial cells. The goblet cell density and mucin component are reduced in Vitamin A deficiency and contact lens use.[35] The lipid component is important for stabilizing the tear film and preventing rapid evaporation. It is produced mainly by the meibomian glands, which are located along the eyelid margin within the tarsal plates.[36] Clear oil secretions are liquid at body temperature, with a melting range of 10°C to 40°C.[37,38] Meibomian gland disease and subsequent malfunction of the lipid component is probably the most common cause of DED.[39] Dysfunction of the tear film presents as a rapid tear break-up time (Figure 2-2). Hyperosmolarity results from reduced aqueous production or increased aqueous evaporation. Tear osmolarity correlates with dry eye severity,[40] and it has been suggested that tear hyperosmolarity is the primary cause of discomfort, ocular surface damage, and inflammation in dry eye.[12,41-44] The levels of various cytokines and proinflammatory molecules including interleukin (IL)-1β, IL-6, IL-16, IL-33, granulocyte colony-stimulating factor (G-CSF), and transforming growth factor (TGF)-α are higher in patients with DED and are correlated with the clinical severity as well.[45]

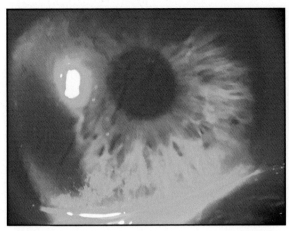

Figure 2-2. This patient has a rapid tear break-up time and dense band of superficial epitheliopathy involving the interpalpebral ocular surface. Her history revealed that she had Sjögren syndrome and spent 8 hours in front of a computer every day.

Conjunctiva

The conjunctiva lines the globe and orbit (bulbar conjunctiva) and the eyelid (palpebral conjunctiva) and contributes to the aqueous and mucous components of tears.[46] Goblet cells account for 5% to 10% of conjunctival epithelial basal cells and are the primary source of mucin in the tear film.[47] The density of goblet cells is influenced by local ocular disease, such as ocular pemphigoid, Stevens-Johnson syndrome, Vitamin A deficiency, and chemical injuries, and by factors in the external environment, such as humidity, temperature, and pollution.[48-50]

Cornea

The cornea maintains its smooth surface through epithelial turnover and neural regulation. The deepest and only mitotically active layer of the corneal epithelium, the basal cells, divide and differentiate into wing cells, which ultimately differentiate into the superficial cells that comprise the layer closest to the surface.[39] The differentiation process takes about 7 to 14 days, after which the superficial cells are desquamated into the tear film.[51] Pathogenic factors such as hypoxia or mechanical stress can induce apoptosis and desquamation of corneal epithelial cells at a rate faster than their maturation, leading to epitheliopathy (Figure 2-3).[52,53]

Loss of corneal sensation results in breakdown of the normal integrity of the cornea, frequently observed as persistent corneal epithelial defects or delayed epithelial wound healing, such as those infected with herpes simplex or herpes zoster viruses, those with advanced diabetes mellitus, and topical anesthetic abuse.[54] Severing corneal nerves with corneal incisions can decrease sensitivity, reflex tear production, and epithelial healing. Corneal nerves, branches of the trigeminal nerve, are the afferent arms of reflex tear production, triggered by cold thermoreceptors, and the involuntary blink response, triggered by polymodal nociceptors (pain receptors). Stimulation of the corneal cold thermoreceptors, leading to increased tear production, show a rise in their firing frequency in a hyperosmolar environment, augmenting tear production.[55] Anesthetized

Figure 2-3. Whorl-like epitheliopathy can be seen when epithelial cell turnover demand outpaces normal cell division in times of stress.

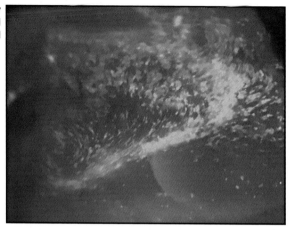

Figure 2-4. The vicious cycle of DED/DTS. The cycle can be initiated at any point. Inflammation and hyperosmolarity result from the effects of DED and serve to further propagate it. MGD = meibomian gland dysfunction. (Adapted from Milner MS, Beckman KA, Luchs JI, et al. Dysfunctional tear syndrome: dry eye disease and associated tear film disorders: new strategies for diagnosis and treatment. *Curr Opin Ophthalmol.* 2017;27[Suppl 1]:3-47.)

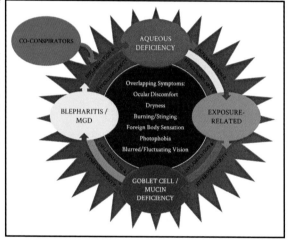

eyes have been shown to have a decreased spontaneous blink rate.[56] Corneal epithelial proliferation is also directly promoted by neuronal interactions through expression of various signaling molecules, which may contribute to the recovery of corneal epithelial cells during injury.[57]

The Vicious Cycle

The complexity of dealing with DED is due to its frustratingly self-perpetuating nature, which has been described as a "vicious cycle"[58] (Figure 2-4). Inflammation and hyperosmolarity are integral parts of the pathophysiology of DED, as both result from and contribute to the perpetuation of the vicious cycle. For example, a patient with Sjögren syndrome can have aqueous deficiency resulting in ocular surface inflammation and hyperosmolarity. Tear film destabilization, microflora proliferation, and

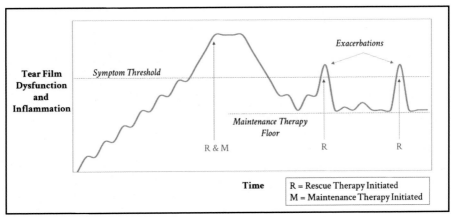

Figure 2-5. DED progression over time.

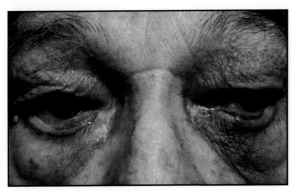

Figure 2-6. For years, this patient treated her chronic symptoms only with lubricating eye drops. Along with Parkinson's disease, her meibomian glands are congested and inflamed and an acute hordeolum is present on the left lower eyelid. The chronic inflammation has led to bilateral ectropia.

inflammatory cell recruitment can develop, causing thickening of meibomian secretions. Obstruction of the glands lead to dysfunction of the lipid component of the tear film and further destabilization, as well as worsening localized eyelid margin inflammation from the retained secretions. As the inflammation turns chronic, the structural components of the eyelids can deteriorate, leading to malposition, exposure, and worsening ocular surface desiccation. The cycle can be entered and initiated at any point, leading to increased inflammation, signs, and symptoms of DED over time.

Figure 2-5 is a graphical representation of the course of a patient with DED. Signs of tear film dysfunction and inflammation accumulate over time until a certain threshold is breached, creating chronic symptoms. Without intervention, the signs and symptoms will continue to worsen. Both rescue and maintenance therapies targeting the specific etiologies are necessary to break the cycle and maintain the level of dryness and inflammation below the threshold of signs and symptoms. The disease state might not be completely reversible, however. When treated early enough, adequate therapy can maintain patients below symptomatic levels. In advanced cases, maintaining a symptom-free course can be extremely challenging or impossible (Figure 2-6).

TABLE 2-1

MAIN SUBTYPES OF DRY EYE DISEASE/ DYSFUNCTIONAL TEAR SYNDROME

Aqueous Tear Deficiency	**Exposure Related**
Lacrimal gland dysfunction	Bell's palsy
Neurotrophic corneas	Parkinson's disease
Sjögren syndrome	Ectropion
Blepharitis/Meibomian Gland Dysfunction	Lagophthalmos
	"Focus" activities
Blepharitis	**Co-Conspirators**
Anterior	Medicamentosa
Posterior	Ocular allergy
Goblet Cell/Mucin Deficiency	Mucus fishing syndrome
Stevens-Johnson syndrome	Conjunctivochalasis
Vitamin A deficiency	Floppy eyelid syndrome
Contact lens wear	
Thermal and chemical injuries	

Adapted from Milner MS, Beckman KA, Luchs JI, et al. Dysfunctional tear syndrome: dry eye disease and associated tear film disorders: new strategies for diagnosis and treatment. *Curr Opin Ophthalmol.* 2017;27(Suppl 1):3-47.

CLASSIFICATION OF DRY EYE DISEASE

Four main subtype classifications used by the DTS panel approach are as follows (Table 2-1)[15]:

1. Aqueous deficiency
2. Blepharitis/meibomian gland dysfunction (MGD)
3. Goblet cell/mucin deficiency
4. Exposure related

The presence of multiple subtypes within a patient is common. A fifth category contains conditions labeled as "DTS co-conspirators" that may masquerade as or contribute to the signs and symptoms of DTS.

Aqueous Deficiency

Aqueous deficiency is characterized by a reduction in the aqueous component of the tear film, mainly formed by secretions from the lacrimal gland. The reduction in the aqueous secretions may be due to dysfunction or destruction of the lacrimal gland or its ductules, which prohibits the aqueous secretions from reaching the ocular surface, resulting in a reduced tear lake and hyperosmolarity.[59-61] A further subclassification is defined according to the presence or absence of a diagnosis of the patient with Sjögren syndrome.[62,63] Sjögren syndrome is a chronic autoimmune disorder characterized by immune cell infiltration of exocrine glands, like the lacrimal and salivary glands, and systemic manifestations due to autoantibody production, immune complex deposition, and lymphocytic infiltration of other organs.[64] Through a similar autoimmune mechanism, severe dry eye is a common finding after allogeneic hematopoietic stem cell transplantation in the form of graft-versus-host disease.[65] Aqueous tear deficiency is a less-frequently occurring etiology than others.[66]

Blepharitis/Meibomian Gland Dysfunction

In 2011, the International Workshop on Meibomian Gland Dysfunction defined MGD as "a common disorder that may be asymptomatic or give rise to symptoms, either confined to the affected eyelids, or arising from MGD-related ocular surface disease, including evaporative dry eye; it can also exacerbate aqueous deficiency dry eye."[67] Anterior blepharitis affects the skin of the eyelid, eyelashes, and eyelash follicles. Posterior blepharitis affects the meibomian glands and meibomian gland orifices.

Causes of anterior blepharitis include seborrheic, atopic, staphylococcal, herpetic, parasitic (ie, *Demodex*), and fungal etiologies. Combinations of the subtypes of blepharitis may occur simultaneously in patients.[68,69] The overgrowth of staphylococcal or other bacteria on the eyelid margin may result in erythema, scaling, and crusting, with folliculitis, collarettes, or pustules present at the base of the eyelashes.[70]

Posterior blepharitis is caused by MGD, commonly characterized by terminal duct obstruction and/or qualitative/quantitative changes in the glandular secretions.[71] Meibum, which is released from the meibomian glands present in the upper and lower eyelids and assisted by the blinking process, creates a thin oily layer over the aqueous component of the tear film, thereby reducing evaporation. Alterations in the nature or quality of meibum may result in a rapid tear break-up time, exposing the ocular surface to desiccating stress.[72,73] Alterations in the posterior eyelid margin, including the development of prominent blood vessels or telangiectasias, thickened or turbid secretions of the meibomian glands, and plugged gland orifices, are primary characteristics of MGD (Figure 2-7).[74] This is one of the most common forms of DED with signs of MGD present in 86% of a mixed patient population with dry eye.[66]

Goblet Cell/Mucin Deficiency

Patients with goblet cell loss suffer from a subsequent reduction in mucin production.[75] Mucin glycoproteins attached to cell membranes interact with soluble mucins in the aqueous component to affect the surface tension of the tear film and improve the spreading of tears. Goblet cell loss and/or mucin deficiency affects the stability of the tear film. Although a rapid tear break-up time is frequently observed in patients with MGD, it is also observed in patients with goblet cell loss and/or mucin deficiency.[49,76,77]

Goblet cell deficiency may result from or be associated with cicatricial conjunctivitis, such as Stevens-Johnson syndrome, toxic epidermal necrolysis, pemphigoid, thermal

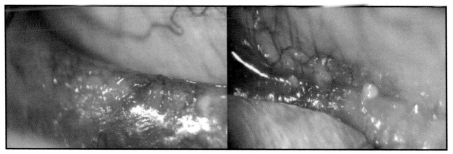

Figure 2-7. Manually expressing thick meibomian secretions. Severe eyelid margin hyperemia and telangiectasias suggest the presence of retained meibomian gland secretions.

and chemical injuries, Vitamin A deficiency, and even epidemic keratoconjunctivitis. Additionally, patients who habitually administer multiple ocular medications, such as glaucoma drops, or those with a history of contact lens use may experience goblet cell loss.[78,79] Vitamin A deficiency affects a substantial number of children and pregnant/lactating women particularly in developing countries.[80] Gastric bypass procedures can cause Vitamin A deficiency leading to serious ocular complications, including xerophthalmia, nyctalopia, and ultimately blindness. The increasing incidence of obesity and gastric bypass procedures warrants patient and physician education regarding strict adherence to vitamin supplementation.[81]

Exposure Related

Excessive drying of the ocular surface due to anatomic defects, improper functioning, or malposition of the eyelids may result in exposure-related DTS. Failure of the eyelids to fully close or abnormal eyelid positioning exposes portions of the ocular surface to the external environment for an extended duration.[82] Exposure of the ocular surface beyond a normal interblink interval can initiate or exacerbate dysfunction of the tear film.[83,84]

Patients with Bell's palsy, Parkinson's disease, or other neurologic disorders may exhibit an incomplete or partial blink. In neurotrophic corneas, a blink reflex can be severely impaired. Even in the absence of apparent exophthalmos, Graves' disease is associated with reduced corneal sensitivity.[85] Situational dry eye occurs when attention to a task, such as driving, reading, or viewing television or hand-held devices, suppresses the blink reflex.[86] Lagophthalmos may be associated with complications resulting from blepharoplasty, scarring of the eyelid, and thyroid eye disease.[87]

Dysfunctional Tear Syndrome Co-Conspirators

The term *co-conspirators* was proposed by the DTS panel to refer to conditions affecting the tear film and ocular surface that may masquerade or exacerbate DTS. These include superior limbic keratoconjunctivitis, Thygeson's superficial punctate keratitis, mucus fishing syndrome, contact lens related toxicity, chemical toxicity, allergic/atopic conjunctivitis, conjunctivochalasis, floppy eyelid syndrome, and corneal hyperalgesia. Medicamentosa is a commonly found co-conspirator with topical antiglaucoma drugs frequently implicated.[88] Complications of skin and eye products can be related to allergy or toxicity.[89] It might be difficult to differentiate these co-conspirators from 1 or more of the 4 main subtypes of DTS, but undiagnosed and untreated DTS co-conspirators can exacerbate and perpetuate DED.[15]

SUMMARY

The definition of DED has evolved over time. Its most recent iteration defines it as "a multifactorial disease of the ocular surface characterized by a loss of homeostasis of the tear film, and accompanied by ocular symptoms, in which tear film instability and hyperosmolarity, ocular surface inflammation and damage, and neurosensory abnormalities play etiological roles."[16] Dysfunction of the lacrimal glands, eyelids, meibomian glands, tear film, conjunctiva, and cornea lead to inflammation and hyperosmolarity of the ocular surface, propagating a vicious cycle that causes worsening signs and symptoms over time. DED can be classified as aqueous deficiency, blepharitis or MGD, goblet cell or mucin deficiency, or exposure related, often with more than one class present in a symptomatic patient.

REFERENCES

1. Duke-Elder WS. Keratitis sicca. *Br J Ophthalmol.* 1930;14(2):61-65.
2. Coppez. Un cas d'absence congénitale de la secretion lacrymale. *Rev. gén. d'Ophtal.*, T. 341, 1920.
3. Wagenmann. *Ber. vers. ophthal. Ges., Heidelberg,* S.172, 1893.
4. Wagenmann. Einiges ueber die Erkrankung der Tränenorgane besonders auch der Tränendrüsen. Münch. med. Wochenschr., Bd. XVI, S. 682, 1902.
5. Fuchs A. Funktionstörung der Speichel und Tränendrüsen. *Ophthal. Ges., Wien,* 1919.
6. Mathews PM, Ramulu PY, Swenor BS, Utine CA, Rubin GS, Akpek EK. Functional impairment of reading in patients with dry eye. *Br J Ophthalmol.* 2017;101(4):481-486.
7. Tounaka K, Yuki K, Kouyama K, et al. Dry eye disease is associated with deterioration of mental health in male Japanese university staff. *Exp Med.* 2014;233(3):215-220.
8. Galor A, Zheng DD, Arheart KL, et al. Dry eye medication use and expenditures: data from the medical expenditure panel survey 2001 to 2006. *Cornea.* 2012;31(12):1403-1407.
9. Chan CC, Crowston JG, Tan R, Marin M, Charles S. Burden of ocular surface disease in patients with glaucoma from Australia. *Asia Pac J Ophthalmol (Phila).* 2013;2(2):79-87.
10. Asbell PA, Spiegel S. Ophthalmologist perceptions regarding treatment of moderate-to-severe dry eye: results of a physician survey. *Eye Contact Lens.* 2010;36(1):33-38.
11. Lemp MA. Report of the National Eye Institute/Industry workshop on clinical trials in dry eyes. *CLAO J.* 1995;21:221-232.
12. Report of the International Dry Eye WorkShop (2007). *Ocul Surf.* 2007;5:69-204.
13. Cornea/External Disease Preferred Practice Pattern Panel. Dry Eye Syndrome PPP—2013. https://www.aao.org/preferred-practice-pattern/dry-eye-syndrome-ppp--2013. Accessed February 2, 2017.
14. Behrens A, Doyle JJ, Stern L, et al., Dysfunctional Tear Syndrome Study Group. Dysfunctional tear syndrome: a Delphi approach to treatment recommendations. *Cornea.* 2006;25:900-907.
15. Milner MS, Beckman KA, Luchs JI, et al. Dysfunctional tear syndrome: dry eye disease and associated tear film disorders: new strategies for diagnosis and treatment. *Curr Opin Ophthalmol.* 2017;27(Suppl 1):3-47.

16. Bron AJ, de Paiva CS, Chauhan SK, et al. TFOS DEWS II pathophysiology report. *Ocul Surf.* 2017;15(3):438-510.

17. Allansmith MR, Kajiyama G, Abelson MB, Simon MA. Plasma cell content of main and accessory lacrimal glands and conjunctiva. *Am J Ophthalmol.* 1976;82(6):819-826.

18. Dartt DA. Neural regulation of lacrimal gland secretory processes: relevance in dry eye diseases. *Prog Retin Eye Res.* 2009;28(3):155-177.

19. Dartt DA. Signal transduction and control of lacrimal gland protein secretion: a review. *Curr Eye Res.* 1989;8(6):619-636.

20. Botelho SY. Tears and the lacrimal gland. *Sci Am.* 1964;211:78-86.

21. Hodges RR, Dartt DA. Regulatory pathways in lacrimal gland epithelium. *Int Rev Cytol.* 2003;231:129-196.

22. Gupta A, Heigle T, Pflugfelder SC. Nasolacrimal stimulation of aqueous tear production. *Cornea.* 1997;16(6):645-648.

23. Wieczorek R, Jakobiec FA, Sacks EH, Knowles DM. The immunoarchitecture of the normal human lacrimal gland. Relevancy for understanding pathologic conditions. *Ophthalmology.* 1988;95(1):100-109.

24. Zoukhri D. Effect of inflammation on lacrimal gland function. *Exp Eye Res.* 2006;82(5):885-898.

25. Kakizaki H, Zako M, Miyashi O, et al. The lacrimal canaliculus and sac bordered by the Horner's muscle form the functional lacrimal drainage system. *Ophthalmology.* 2005;112(4):710-716.

26. Tsubota K. Tear dynamics and dry eye. *Prog Retin Eye Res.* 1998;17(4):565-596.

27. Alex A, Edwards A, Hays JD, et al. Factors predicting the ocular surface response to desiccating environmental stress. *Invest Ophthalmol Vis Sci.* 2013;54(5):3325-3332.

28. Moore QL, De Paiva CS, Pflugfelder SC. Effects of dry eye therapies on environmentally induced ocular surface disease. *Am J Ophthalmol.* 2015;160(1):135-142.e1.

29. Ousler GW 3rd, Rodriguez JD, Smith LM, et al. Optimizing reading tests for dry eye disease. *Cornea.* 2015;34(8):917-921.

30. Jansen ME, Begley CG, Himebaugh NH, Port NL. Effect of contact lens wear and a near task on tear film break-up. *Optom Vis Sci.* 2010;87(5):350-357.

31. Tsubota K, Shimmura S, Shinozaki N, Holland EJ, Shimazaki J. Clinical application of living-related conjunctival-limbal allograft. *Am J Ophthalmol.* 2002;133(1):134-135.

32. Lipham WJ, Tawfik HA, Dutton JJ. A histologic analysis and three-dimensional reconstruction of the muscle of Riolan. *Ophthl Plast Reconstr Surg.* 2002;18(2):93-98.

33. Yokoi N, Bron AJ, Tiffany JM, Maruyama K, Komuro A, Kinoshita S. Relationship between tear volume and tear meniscus curvature. *Arch Ophthalmol.* 2004;122(9):1265-1269.

34. Tung CI, Perin AF, Gumus K, Pflugfelder SC. Tear meniscus dimensions in tear dysfunction and their correlation with clinical parameters. *Am J Ophthalmol.* 2014;157(2):301-310.

35. Klyce SD, Beuerman RW. Structure and function of the cornea. In: Kaufman HE, Barron BA, McDonald MB, Waltman SR, eds. *The Cornea.* New York, NY: Churchill Livingstone; 1988:3-54.

36. Colorado LH, Alzahrani Y, Pritchard N, Efron N. Time course of changes in goblet cell density in symptomatic and asymptomatic contact lens wearers. *Invest Ophthalmol Vis Sci.* 2016;57(6):2560-2566.

37. Tiffany JM. The lipid secretion of the meibomian glands. *Adv Lipid Res.* 1987;22:1-62.

38. Butovich IA, Lu H, McMahon A, et al. Biophysical and morphological evaluation of human normal and dry eye meibum using hot stage polarized light microscopy. *Invest Ophthalmol Vis Sci.* 2014;55(1):87-101.

39. Lemp MA, Beuerman RW. Tear film. In: Krachmer JH, Mannis MJ, Holland EJ, eds. *Cornea.* 3rd ed. Beijing, China: Mosby Elsevier; 2011:41-46.

40. Nishida T, Saika S. Cornea and sclera: anatomy and physiology. In: Krachmer JH, Mannis MJ, Holland EJ, eds. *Cornea.* 3rd ed. Beijing, China: Mosby Elsevier; 3-24.

41. Suzuki M, Massingale ML, Ye F, et al. Tear osmolarity as a biomarker for dry eye disease severity. *Invest Ophthalmol Vis Sci.* 2010;51(9):4557-4561.

42. Farris RL, Gilbard JP, Stuchell N, et al. Diagnostic tests in keratoconjunctivitis sicca. *CLAO J.* 1983;9:23-28.

43. Gilbard JP, Farris RL, Santamaria J 2nd. Osmolarity of tear micro volumes in keratoconjunctivitis sicca. *Arch Ophthalmol.* 1978;96:677-681.

44. Gilbard JP, Rossi SR, Gray KL. A new rabbit model for keratoconjunctivitis sicca. *Invest Ophthalmol Vis Sci.* 1987;28:225-228.

45. Gilbard JP, Rossi SR, Gray KL. Tear film and ocular surface changes after closure of the meibomian gland orifices in the rabbit. *Ophthalmology.* 1989;96:1180-1186.

46. Na KS, Mok JW, Kim JY, Rho CR, Joo CK. Correlations between tear cytokines, chemokines, and soluble receptors and clinical severity of dry eye disease. *Invest Ophthalmol Vis Sci.* 2012;53(9):5443-5450.

47. Nelson JD, Cameron JD. The conjunctiva: anatomy and physiology. In: Krachmer JH, Mannis MJ, Holland EJ, eds. *Cornea.* 3rd ed. Beijing, China: Mosby Elsevier; 25-31.

48. Thoft R, Friend J. Ocular surface evaluation. In: Francois J, Brown S, Itoi M, eds. Proceedings of the symposium of the International Society for Corneal Research. Doc Ophthalmol Proc Series 20. The Hague, The Netherlands; 1980.

49. Nelson JD, Wright JC. Conjunctival goblet cell densities in ocular surface disease. *Arch Ophthalmol.* 1984;102(7):1049-1051.

50. Ralph RA. Conjunctival goblet cell density in normal subjects and in dry eye syndromes. *Invest Ophthalmol.* 1975;14(4):299-302.

51. Waheed MA, Basu PK. The effect of air pollutants on the eye. I. The effect of an organic extract on the conjunctival goblet cells. *Can J Ophthalmol.* 1970;5(3):226-230.

52. Hanna C, Bicknell DS, O'Brien JE. Cell turnover in the adult human eye. *Arch Ophthalmol.* 1961;65:695-698.

53. Esco MA, Wang Z, McDermott ML, Kurpakus-Wheater M. Potential role for laminin 5 in hypoxia-mediated apoptosis of human corneal epithelial cells. *J Cell Sci.* 2001;114(Pt 22):4033-4040.

54. Li L, Ren DH, Ladage PM, et al. Annexin V binding to rabbit corneal epithelial cells following overnight contact lens wear or eyelid closure. *CLAO J.* 2002;28(1):48-54.

55. Bisla K, Tanelian DL. Concentration-dependent effects of lidocaine on corneal epithelial wound healing. *Invest Ophthalmol Vis Sci.* 1992;33(11):3029-3033.

56. Parra A, Gonzalez-Gonzalez O, Gallar J, Belmonte C. Tear fluid hyperosmolality increases nerve impulse activity of cold thermoreceptor endings of the cornea. *Pain.* 2014;155(8):1481-1491.

57. Borges FP, Garcia DM, Cruz AA. Distribution of spontaneous inter-blink interval in repeated measurements with and without topical ocular anesthesia. *Arq Bras Oftalmol.* 2010;73(4):329-332.

58. Kowtharapu BS, Stahnke T, Wree A, Guthoff RF, Stachs O. Corneal epithelial and neuronal interactions: role in wound healing. *Exp Eye Res.* 2014;125:53-61.

59. Baudouin C, Messmer EM, Aragona P, et al. Revisiting the vicious circle of dry eye disease: a focus on the pathophysiology of meibomian gland dysfunction. *Br J Ophthalmol.* 2016;100(3):300-306.

60. Mishima S, Gasset A, Klyce SD Jr, Baum JL. Determination of tear volume and tear flow. *Invest Ophthalmol.* 1966;5:264-276.

61. Scherz W, Dohlman CH. Is the lacrimal gland dispensable? Keratoconjunctivitis sicca after lacrimal gland removal. *Arch Ophthalmol.* 1975;93:281-283.

62. Li DQ, Chen Z, Song XJ, et al. Stimulation of matrixmetalloproteinases by hyperosmolarity via a JNK pathway in human cornealepithelial cells. *Invest Ophthalmol Vis Sci.* 2004;45:4302-4311.

63. Lemp MA, Crews LA, Bron AJ, et al. Distribution of aqueous-deficient and evaporative dry eye in a clinic-based patient cohort: a retrospective study. *Cornea.* 2012;31:472-478.

64. Thompson N, Isenberg DA, Jury EC, Ciurtin C. Exploring BAFF: its expression, receptors and contribution to the immunopathogenesis of Sjögren's syndrome. *Rheumatology (Oxford).* 2016;55(9):1548-1555.

65. Damato BE, Allan D, Murray SB, Lee WR. Senile atrophy of the human lacrimal gland: the contribution of chronic inflammatory disease. *Br J Ophthalmol.* 1984;68:674-680.

66. Ivanir Y, Shimoni A, Ezra-Nimni O, Barequet IS. Prevalence of dry eye syndrome after allogeneic hematopoietic stem cell transplantation. *Cornea.* 2013;32(5):e97-e101.

67. Martinez JD, Galor A, Ramos-Betancourt N, et al. Frequency and risk factors associated with dry eye in patients attending a tertiary care ophthalmology center in Mexico City. *Clin Ophthalmol.* 2016;10:1335-1342.

68. Nichols KK, Foulks GN, Bron AJ, et al. The International Workshop on Meibomian Gland Dysfunction. *Invest Ophthalmol Vis Sci.* 2011;52:1917-2085.

69. McCulley JP, Dougherty JM, Deneau DG. Classification of chronic blepharitis. *Ophthalmology.* 1982;89:1173-1180.

70. Jackson WB. Blepharitis: current strategies for diagnosis and management. *Can J Ophthalmol.* 2008;43:170-179.

71. Arita R, Fukuoka S, Morishige N. New Insights into the lipid layer of the tear film and meibomian glands. *Eye Contact Lens.* 2017;43(6):335-339.
72. Nichols KK, Foulks GN, Bron AJ, et al. The International Workshop on Meibomian Gland Dysfunction: executive summary. *Invest Ophthalmol Vis Sci.* 2011;52(4):1922-1929.
73. Shine WE, McCulley JP. The role of cholesterol in chronic blepharitis. *Invest Ophthalmol Vis Sci.* 1991;32:2272-2280.
74. Shine WE, Silvany R, McCulley JP. Relation of cholesterol-stimulated *Staphylococcus aureus* growth to chronic blepharitis. *Invest Ophthalmol Vis Sci.* 1993;34:2291-2296.
75. McCulley JP, Shine WE. Meibomian secretions in chronic blepharitis. *Adv Exp Med Biol.* 1998;438:319-326.
76. Bowling B. *Kanski's Clinical Ophthalmology: A Systematic Approach.* 8th ed. Cambridge, MA: Elsevier; 2016.
77. Pflugfelder SC, Tseng SC, Yoshino K, et al. Correlation of goblet cell density and mucosal epithelial membrane mucin expression with rose Bengal staining in patients with ocular irritation. *Ophthalmology.* 1997;104:223-235.
78. Tei M, Spurr-Michaud SJ, Tisdale AS, Gipson IK. Vitamin A deficiency alters the expression of mucin genes by the rat ocular surface epithelium. *Invest Ophthalmol Vis Sci.* 2000;41:82-88.
79. Kunert KS, Tisdale AS, Gipson IK. Goblet cell numbers and epithelial proliferation in the conjunctiva of patients with dry eye syndrome treated with cyclosporine. *Arch Ophthalmol.* 2002;120:330-337.
80. Doughty MJ. Contact lens wear and the goblet cells of the human conjunctiva: a review. *Cont Lens Anterior Eye.* 2011;34:157-163.
81. Akhtar S, Ahmed A, Randhawa MA, et al. Prevalence of vitamin A deficiency in South Asia: causes, outcomes, and possible remedies. *J Health Popul Nutr.* 2013;31(4):413-423.
82. Lee WB, Hamilton SM, Harris JP, Schwab IR. Ocular complications of hypovitaminosis a after bariatric surgery. *Ophthalmology.* 2005;112(6):1031-1034.
83. Lemp MA. Breakup of the tear film. *Int Ophthalmol Clin.* 1973;13:97-102.
84. Tsubota K, Nakamori K. Effects of ocular surface area and blink rate on tear dynamics. *Arch Ophthalmol.* 1995;113:155-158.
85. Abelson MB, Ousler GW 3rd, Nally LA, et al. Alternative reference values for tear film breakup time in normal and dry eye populations. *Adv Exp Med Biol.* 2002;506:1121-1125.
86. Achtsidis V, Tentolouris N, Theodoropoulou S, et al. Dry eye in Graves ophthalmopathy: correlation with corneal hypoesthesia. *Eur J Ophthalmol.* 2013;23(4):473-479.
87. Moon JH, Kim KW, Moon NJ. Smartphone use is a risk factor for pediatric dry eye disease according to region and age: a case control study. *BMC Ophthalmol.* 2016;16(1):188.
88. Latkany RL, Lock B, Speaker M. Nocturnal lagophthalmos: an overview and classification. *Ocul Surf.* 2006;4:44-53.
89. Aydin Kurna S, Acikgoz S, Altun A, Ozbay N, Sengor T, Olcaysu OO. The effects of topical antiglaucoma drugs as monotherapy on the ocular surface: a prospective study. *J Ophthalmol.* 2014;2014:460-483.

SECTION II

EXAMINATION AND DIAGNOSTICS

CHAPTER 3

Ocular Surface Disease Index and Patient History

Nandini Venkateswaran, MD and Anat Galor, MD, MSPH

KEY POINTS

- Dry eye disease (DED) can manifest variably among patients. Presenting symptoms are numerous, ranging from foreign body sensation, irritation, and pain to profound photophobia and blurred vision.
- There is no gold standard test to diagnose DED. Patient symptomatology is important in the management of DED because clinical findings often underestimate the severity of symptoms and their impact on patient quality of life.
- Subjective questionnaires that record and quantify symptoms have emerged as practical tools for the diagnosis and management of DED.

Dry eye disease (DED) is traditionally defined as a multifactorial disease of the tears and ocular surface, but it is also predominantly a symptomatic disease.[1] DED can manifest variably among patients and presenting symptoms are numerous, ranging from foreign body sensation, irritation, and pain to profound photophobia and blurred vision.[2] Multiple testing modalities are employed to evaluate the ocular surface in patients with symptoms of DED, including tear osmolarity testing, tear break-up time, fluorescein

Mah FS, Rhee MK, eds.
Dry Eye Disease: A Practical Guide (pp 27-38).
© 2019 Taylor & Francis Group.

staining, lissamine green staining, Schirmer testing type 1 and 2, among others; however, there is no gold standard test to diagnose DED.[1,2] In fact, ophthalmologists often rely heavily on patient history and symptomatology to help guide their clinical thought process as, often, clinical findings underestimate the severity of DED symptoms and their impact on patients' quality of life.[3-5] Subjective questionnaires that record and quantify symptoms have emerged as practical tools for the diagnosis and management of DED.[3,4] In this chapter, we discuss the role of a thorough patient history as well as patient questionnaires in the diagnosis and management of DED.

PATIENT HISTORY

According to the American Academy of Ophthalmology Preferred Practice Guidelines in 2013, a detailed patient history is critical in eliciting important information.[6] The history should include a description of the patient's signs and symptoms, duration of signs and symptoms, exacerbating conditions, as well as a thorough ocular and medical history.

DED symptoms that patients can report include a wide range of dysesthesias often characterized as dryness, irritation, burning, tenderness, and aching, to name a few, as well as visual complaints such as blurred or fluctuating vision, tearing, and/or contact lens intolerance. Exacerbating conditions can include changes in environmental conditions such as air travel, changes in humidity, and exposure to wind and light, as well as activities inducing reduced blink rates such as reading and computer use. A comprehensive ocular history should investigate prior ocular surgery (eg, refractive surgery), prior eyelid or punctal surgery, prior facial palsies or ocular surface disease, topical or systemic medication use, and contact lens use and hygiene. A comprehensive medical history should explore dermatological diseases, systemic inflammatory diseases, neurological conditions, chronic pain conditions, sleep disorders (eg, sleep apnea and continuous positive airway pressure treatment), atopic disease, prior malignancies requiring radiation of the orbit, hormonal changes, chronic viral infections, trauma, mental health disorders, and use of systemic medications (such as antihistamines, antidepressants, diuretics, hormone replacement, cardiac medications, and chemotherapeutic agents). The ability to address all aspects of a patient history can be difficult in a short office visit and many times physicians use questionnaires to help complete a thorough patient history.[3]

TYPES OF QUESTIONNAIRES

There are several validated questionnaires that can be used in the clinical setting to assess DED. In 2007, the International Dry Eye WorkShop published a report on the epidemiology of dry eye that evaluated the utility of a number of dry eye questionnaires in diagnosing DED.[1] They determined several characteristics of dry eye questionnaires that contributed to the suitability for use of these tools in epidemiologic studies and randomized controlled trials. These characteristics included[1]:

- Ability to detect and measure a change in symptoms with effective treatment or disease progression
- Ability to detect therapeutic response by a drug
- Ability to be reproducible
- Have a specified recall period
- Ability to set a threshold of severity of disease as an inclusion criteria

Although these characteristics were primarily for the use of questionnaires for research studies, they can certainly be applied to clinical practice. Clinicians aim to implement validated, reliable dry eye questionnaires that accurately assesses patient symptoms and quality of life measures and assist them in diagnosing and managing DED.[3,4]

THE OCULAR SURFACE DISEASE INDEX QUESTIONNAIRE

The Ocular Surface Disease Index (OSDI) was one of the validated questionnaires highlighted in the International Dry Eye WorkShop report and is one of the most frequently used instruments to evaluate DED.[1] First introduced in 1997 by the Outcomes Research Group by Allergan Inc, the questionnaire has been employed to assess the symptoms of DED and their impact on vision-related functioning. The questionnaire initially contained 40 items but was condensed to 12 items after psychometric analyses examined its validity and reliability in a clinical trial. The questionnaire consists of 12 questions that evaluate the presence of ocular symptoms of DED, the timing and frequency of symptoms over the preceding week when performing vision-related activities, and the occurrence of symptoms with certain environmental triggers. Each question has a 5-category Likert-type response option, ranging from "none of the time" to "all the time." An option of "not applicable" is available for patients who did not perform the activities or experience any of the vision-related functions and environmental conditions outlined. The questionnaire requires approximately 5 minutes to complete and is scored from 0 to 100 points, with symptoms categorized as normal (0 to 12), mild DED (13 to 22), moderate DED (23 to 32), or severe DED (33 to 100).[6,7]

The OSDI has undergone extensive reliability testing since its inception. Schiffman et al conducted a study in 2000 to evaluate the validity and reliability of the OSDI questionnaire in a sample of patients with DED and normal controls. In this study, the Cronbach alpha, a measure of internal consistency, exceeded 0.7 and ranged from good to excellent for the overall instrument as well as for 3 subscales (ocular symptoms, vision-related function, and environmental triggers). Test-retest reliability was also good to excellent, suggesting that questionnaire results were reproducible. The OSDI was also effective in discriminating normal, mild to moderate, and severe DED, as determined by physician assessment as well as a composite disease severity score. OSDI scores also correlated well with other eye-specific health status measures, including the McMonnies, National Eye Institute Visual Functioning, and Short-Form 12 Health questionnaires. Overall, this study illustrated that the OSDI was a valid and reliable instrument to assess DED.[8]

There are certain limitations to the OSDI questionnaire. The questionnaire addresses only a handful of dry eye symptoms, such as photophobia, grittiness, pain, and blurred vision. It explores the effect of DED on vision-related function as well as the effect of environmental triggers on symptoms but only highlights certain activities and triggers. It investigates the frequency of symptoms over the preceding week but does not directly measure severity nor the temporal course of the disease. As such, while the questionnaire is short and straightforward to complete, it only partially captures the effects of DED on patient quality of life.[3] The study by Schiffman et al also found that the questionnaire only weakly correlated with clinical dry eye tests,[8] an outcome replicated by several groups using different questionnaires.[9-11] Another limitation of the OSDI is the compilation of all responses into one total score, despite the reality that different biological mechanisms underlie different items. For example, OSDI items that ask about spontaneous pain in the form of "gritty" or "sore eyes" point to nerve stimulation, while those that ask about visual complaints point to ocular surface pathology. Furthermore, certain pain complaints, such as evoked pain to wind and light, point to a neuropathic etiology.[12,13]

In general, pain is categorized by the status of the nociceptive system; pain transmitted through an intact system is referred to as *nociceptive* while pain transmitted through an abnormal system is referred to as *neuropathic*.[14] In the eye, nociceptive pain refers to pain induced by an abnormal ocular surface environment (high osmolarity, decreased tear volume, increase evaporation rate) in the setting of an intact system. Neuropathic pain, on the other hand, refers to pain that is transmitted by altered or sensitized system. In DED, nerve sensitization can occur for many reasons, including high tear osmolarity, ocular surface inflammation, trauma, and/or genetic predisposition, with resultant changes in nerve behavior (ie, nerves that fire spontaneously or at lower thresholds). As such, focusing on responses to individual items within the OSDI may help tailor the diagnosis and treatment of DED, including identifying patients more likely to have neuropathic ocular pain.[13]

Ngo et al[15] recently conducted a prospective study to determine if OSDI scores differed when the questionnaire was taken independently or with examiner guidance. The study found that there was no significant difference in the OSDI score between the 2 groups; however, examiner guidance did affect the variability of scores in the older group, which consisted of patients over 45 years old. As such, while many patients in the office setting can take this questionnaire independently, a certain subset of patients may benefit from guidance when completing the questionnaire, leading to more accurate results. However, the length and design of the questionnaire allows it to be an easy tool to employ in the outpatient ophthalmology setting.[15]

OTHER AVAILABLE QUESTIONNAIRES

There are several other validated questionnaires in addition to the OSDI that are employed for the assessment of DED. These include the Dry Eye Questionnaire-5 (DEQ-5), McMonnies Questionnaire (MQ), Impact of Dry Eye on Everyday Life (IDEEL) Questionnaire, National Eye Institute Visual Functioning Questionnaire-25

(NEI VFQ-25), Standard Patient Evaluation of Eye Dryness (SPEED) Questionnaire, and Symptom Assessment in Dry Eye (SANDE) Questionnaire.[1] We have created a table that highlights the overall features of 6 of these different questionnaires and provide brief descriptions (Table 3-1).

The DEQ-5 questionnaire was created by Chalmers, Begley, and Caffery and consists of 5 questions that are used to distinguish patients with and without DED. Scores range from 0 to 22 with higher scores being more indicative of DED. The questionnaire primarily focuses on pain complaints, including presence and intensity of dryness, eye discomfort, and eye watering. It importantly does not include questions on vision complaints, functional status, or quality of life measures, which limits its ability to assess the effect of DED on visual function.[16] However, in an older population with frequent visual complaints, focusing on the pain complaints of DED may be more appropriate. As it is difficult to tease out in a questionnaire the etiology behind "poor vision" (ie, DED vs other ocular pathology), scores on the OSDI may be artificially high for reasons other than DED in older populations.

The MQ developed by McMonnies and Ho consists of 12 questions. The questionnaire assesses pain complaints, such as dryness, grittiness, soreness, burning, and irritation on waking, as well as evoked pain to cigarette smoke, smog, air conditioning, heating, swimming, and alcohol use. Scores range from 0 to 45 with higher scores indicative of higher DED symptoms. Similar to the DEQ-5, vision complaints, functional assessments, and quality of life measures are not directly addressed, but the questionnaire does ask about previous and current DED treatment, comorbid systemic conditions such as thyroid disease, arthritis, or mucous membrane dryness, as well as medication use. These questions permit physicians to augment their patient history and investigate comorbidities that can contribute to DED.[17]

The IDEEL questionnaire developed by Alcon consists of 57 questions comprised of 3 modules: Dry Eye Symptom Bother, Dry Eye Impact on Daily Life, and Dry Eye Treatment Satisfaction. Within the Daily Life and Treatment Satisfaction modules there are subscales:

- Impact on daily activities, emotional impact, and impact on work within the daily life module
- Satisfaction with treatment effectiveness and treatment-related bother/inconvenience in the treatment satisfaction module

The questionnaire covers multiple domains of DED, including symptoms such as itching burning, dryness, swelling, redness, as well as functional and quality of life domains (including vision function and psychological, social, and cognitive aspects). Unlike other questionnaires discussed here, patients are also asked about their treatment satisfaction in attempts to monitor progression and improvement. Each module is scored from 0 to 100. Higher scores indicate worse DED symptoms, better quality of life, and better treatment satisfaction.[18] A downside of the questionnaire is its length, which makes both completion and scoring time consuming. As such, it is generally used in research studies and not in the clinical arena.

The National Eye Institute developed the NEI VFQ-25 questionnaire to measure vision-related functioning experienced by patients with various chronic eye diseases.[19] The questions are grouped into 12 subscales that include general health, general vision,

TABLE 3-1

QUESTIONNAIRE CHARACTERISTICS				
NAME OF QUESTIONNAIRE	**NUMBER OF QUESTIONS**	**PAIN COMPLAINTS**	**VISUAL COMPLAINTS**	
OSDI	12	Sensitivity to light, grittiness, pain, soreness, discomfort, environmental triggers (wind, low humidity, air conditioning)	Blurred vision, poor vision	
DEQ-5	5	Discomfort, dryness, watering	N/A	
McMonnies	12	Dryness, grittiness, soreness, tiredness, burning, irritation on waking, triggers (smoke, smog, air conditioning, heating, swimming, alcohol)	N/A	
IDEEL	57; 3 modules	Grittiness, sandy, burning, stinging, itching, irritation, scratchiness, dryness, mucus, puffy and swollen, redness, aching, soreness	Blurry vision, eye tiredness	
NEI VFQ-25	25; 12 subscales	Burning, itching, aching	Quality of eyesight	
SPEED	4	Dryness, grittiness, scratchiness, soreness, irritation, burning, watering	Eye fatigue	
SANDE	2	Dryness and irritation	N/A	

*higher scores indicate worse symptoms.
†higher scores indicate worse symptoms, but better quality of life and treatment satisfaction.

QUESTIONNAIRE CHARACTERISTICS

FUNCTIONAL ASSESSMENTS	QUALITY OF LIFE ASSESSMENTS	ADDITIONAL QUESTIONS	SCORING
Limitations in reading, driving at night, working with computer or ATM, watching television	N/A	N/A	0 to 100*
N/A	N/A	N/A	0 to 22*
N/A	N/A	Previous and current treatment, systemic arthritis or thyroid disease, mucous membrane dryness, medications, lagophthalmos	0 to 45*
Doing close work, doing work in dimly-lit conditions, driving, working on the computer, being in areas with scented products or smoke	Daily activity limitations, impact on work, emotional well-being	Treatment satisfaction	Each module 0 to 100†
Difficulty with a range of activities requiring near vision and distance vision	Quality of general health and general vision, limitations in ability to work, limitations in social function, effect on mental health	N/A	Each subscale 0 to 100 along with a combined total score from 0 to 100*
N/A	N/A	N/A	0 to 28*
N/A	N/A	N/A	√ (frequency x severity)

ocular pain, near activities, distance activities, social functioning, mental health, role difficulties, dependency, driving, color vision, and peripheral vision. Within the ocular pain subscale, symptoms such as pain, eye discomfort, burning, itching, and aching are included. Each subscale is scored from 0 to 100, and a combined total score is also generated, where higher scores indicate more vision-related disability. One of the unique aspects of this questionnaire is that it was not created to be condition specific but rather to be employed for various vision problems. Studies have shown that the questionnaire is reliable and valid in assessing the influences of cataract, macular degeneration, glaucomatous field loss, and even DED on vision-related function.[20] This can be perceived as both an advantage, as the questionnaire can be compared across various diseases, but also as a disadvantage, as it may lack the sensitivity of a DED-specific questionnaire. In addition, its length and complexity render it more of a research tool rather than an adjunct in clinical practice. However, if used in the evaluation of DED, the questionnaire, similar to the IDEEL questionnaire, can analyze specific responses within each subscale and helps the physician better identify in which areas a patient is most affected by DED.[21]

The SPEED questionnaire developed by Tear-Science is a frequency- and severity-based questionnaire consisting of 8 questions that tracks diurnal and long-term DED symptom changes over a 3-month period. Scores are summed from the frequency and severity portions of the questionnaire, and the total score can range from 0 to 28, with higher scores suggesting higher frequency and severity of DED symptoms. The questionnaire is able to accurately evaluate the frequency and severity of DED symptoms and distinguish symptomatic from asymptomatic DED patients; however, similar to other questionnaires discussed previously, it does not address functional and quality of life measures.[7]

The SANDE questionnaire developed by TearLab uses a 100-mm linear visual analog scale that quantifies the severity and frequency of dry eye symptoms.[22] The questionnaire only consists of 2 questions, one assessing symptom frequency and the other symptom severity. Frequency options range from "rarely" to "all the time" while severity ranges from "very mild" to "very severe." Patients mark where they fall along this linear scale, and the distance is measured in millimeters. Scores are obtained by obtaining the product of the measurement for frequency of symptoms with the measurements of severity of symptoms and then obtaining the square root. The questionnaire is effective in assessing the presence and severity of DED but does not capture functional assessments as well as quality of life measures related to DED. However, as many patients use different words to describe DED symptoms, this questionnaire has the benefit of incorporating all these different terms under the 2 items.

Given the similarity between DED symptoms and pain complaints elsewhere in the body, researchers have examined whether questionnaires commonly used to diagnose and manage nonocular pain can be applied to the eye.[14,23] For example, a numerical rating scale (NRS) can be used to rate the intensity of pain over variable recall periods using a scale anchored at 0 for "no pain sensation" and at 10 for "the most intense eye pain imaginable." This type of 0 to 10 NRS has been validated as a measure of pain intensity across multiple populations[24-28] and has been recommended for use as the primary outcome metric in clinical trials for chronic pain.[29] Using this questionnaire, individuals who reported DED symptoms were found to also report ocular pain[14]:

- 11% (n = 17) of subjects reported no pain (NRS 0) on average over a 1-week recall period
- 36% (n = 56) reported mild pain (NRS 1 to 3)
- 34% (n = 52) reported moderate pain (NRS 4 to 6)
- 19% (n = 29) reported severe pain (NRS 7 to 10)

Another commonly used questionnaire is the Neuropathic Pain Symptom Inventory (NPSI). The NPSI has been validated as an appropriate self-report instrument for assessing neuropathic pain,[30] has been used to quantify different aspects of neuropathic pain,[31] and has been found to correlate with mechanical/thermal allodynia and hyperalgesia assessed using quantitative sensory testing.[31] The NPSI asks about 7 descriptors that are commonly associated with neuropathic pain (ie, burning, squeezing, pressure, electric shocks, stabbing, pins/needles, tingling). One group studied the use of the questionnaire in DED by altering the questions on evoked pain (items 8, 9, and 10, questions regarding the severity of allodynia or hyperalgesia caused by [1] light touch, [2] pressure, or [3] contact with something cold on the skin) to questions specific to ocular pain (eye pain caused or increased by [1] wind, [2] light, and [3] heat or cold).[32] Using these 10 items, a total NPSI eye score is calculated (range 0 to 100), along with 5 subscores (burning spontaneous pain, pressing spontaneous pain, paroxysmal pain, evoked pain, and paresthesia/dysesthesia). In individuals with DED symptoms, ocular NPSI and NRS scores were found to be well correlated (Pearson $r = 0.66$).[14]

COMPARISON OF QUESTIONNAIRES WITH THE OCULAR SURFACE DISEASE INDEX

Studies in the literature have compared the efficacy of the OSDI questionnaire with other questionnaires. Asiedu et al conducted a cross-sectional study comparing the SPEED and OSDI questionnaires. In a sample of 657 patients, the study found that there was good internal consistency of both questionnaires (Cronbach alpha of 0.895 for SPEED and 0.897 for OSDI) and that there was a significant correlation between the total scores of both ($r = 0.68$).[7] Amparo et al[22] compared patient-reported symptoms of DED as assessed by the OSDI and SANDE. In this study of 114 patients, scores from both questionnaires were significantly correlated both at the baseline visit ($r = 0.64$) as well as between changes in scores from the baseline visit to follow-up visit ($r = 0.47$).[22] In a cross-sectional study of 154 patients with idiopathic DED symptoms, Kalangara et al found good correlations between the DEQ-5 and OSDI (Pearson $r = 0.64$).[14]

These studies illustrate that other validated questionnaires are available to evaluate for DED. However, similar to the OSDI, they each come with their set of disadvantages. Questionnaires vary in length, which may limit which patient population they can be employed in, and assess DED symptoms using different scales making comparability difficult. The majority explore DED symptomatology, while fewer also explore functional limitations and vision related quality of life. The majority of the questionnaires provide one total score; however, questionnaires like IDEEL and NEI VFQ-25 provide scores for each subscale, as mentioned previously. In our opinion, an ideal questionnaire should provide a total score as well as scores of individual metrics to help better understand the pathophysiology of each patient's DED. Differentiating between different subgroups of DED as well as the effects of their symptoms of function and quality of life can be instrumental in individualizing treatment.

SUMMARY

Patient symptom questionnaires are an important adjunct in the diagnosis and management of DED. While there are many questionnaires available, physicians have to ultimately choose the questionnaires he or she feels are best suited for his or her clinical practice. Some questionnaires may be more useful as screening tools, while others can be used to monitor the long-term progression and management of DED. It is important to use questionnaires in conjunction with a thorough patient history, objective testing, and clinical examination to tailor treatment and management plans.

ACKNOWLEDGMENTS

Supported by the Department of Veterans Affairs, Veterans Health Administration, Office of Research and Development, Clinical Sciences Research EPID-006-15S (Dr. Galor), R01EY026174 (Dr. Galor), NIH Center Core Grant P30EY014801, and Research to Prevent Blindness Unrestricted Grant.

REFERENCES

1. The epidemiology of dry eye disease: report of the Epidemiology Subcommittee of the International Dry Eye WorkShop (2007). *Ocul Surf.* 2007;5(2):93-107.
2. McGinnigle S, Naroo SA, Eperjesi F. Evaluation of dry eye. *Surv Ophthalmol.* 2012;57(4):293-316.
3. Grubbs JR Jr, Tolleson-Rinehart S, Huynh K, Davis RM. A review of quality of life measures in dry eye questionnaires. *Cornea.* 2014;33(2):215-218.
4. Friedman NJ. Impact of dry eye disease and treatment on quality of life. *Curr Opin Ophthalmol.* 2010;21(4):310-316.
5. Guillemin I, Begley C, Chalmers R, et al. Appraisal of patient-reported outcome instruments available for randomized clinical trials in dry eye: revisiting the standards. *Ocul Surf.* 2012;10(2):84-99.
6. Cornea/External Disease Preferred Practice Pattern Panel. Dry Eye Syndrome PPP—2013. https://www.aao.org/preferred-practice-pattern/dry-eye-syndrome-ppp--2013. Accessed July 30, 2018.
7. Asiedu K, Kyei S, Mensah SN, et al. Ocular Surface Disease Index (OSDI) versus the Standard Patient Evaluation of Eye Dryness (SPEED): a study of a nonclinical sample. *Cornea.* 2016;35(2):175-180.

8. Schiffman RM, Christianson MD, Jacobsen G, et al. Reliability and validity of the Ocular Surface Disease Index. *Arch Ophthalmol.* 2000;118(5):615-621.

9. Martinez JD, Galor A, Ramos-Betancourt N, et al. Frequency and risk factors associated with dry eye in patients attending a tertiary care ophthalmology center in Mexico City. *Clin Ophthalmol.* 2016;10:1335-1342.

10. Galor A, Feuer W, Lee DJ, et al. Ocular surface parameters in older male veterans. *Invest Ophthalmol Vis Sci.* 2013;54(2):1426-1433.

11. Schein OD, Tielsch JM, Munoz B, et al. Relation between signs and symptoms of dry eye in the elderly. A population-based perspective. *Ophthalmology.* 1997;104(9):1395-1401.

12. Crane AM, Feuer W, Felix ER, et al. Evidence of central sensitisation in those with dry eye symptoms and neuropathic-like ocular pain complaints: incomplete response to topical anaesthesia and generalised heightened sensitivity to evoked pain. *Br J Ophthalmol.* 2017;101(9):1238-1243.

13. Galor A, Levitt RC, Felix ER, et al. Neuropathic ocular pain: an important yet underevaluated feature of dry eye. *Eye (Lond).* 2015;29(3):301-312.

14. Kalangara JP, Galor A, Levitt RC, et al. Characteristics of Ocular Pain Complaints in Patients With Idiopathic Dry Eye Symptoms. *Eye Contact Lens.* 2017;43(3):192-198.

15. Ngo W, Srinivasan S, Keech A, et al. Self versus examiner administration of the Ocular Surface Disease Index. *J Optom.* 2017;10(1):34-42.

16. Chalmers RL, Begley CG, Caffery B. Validation of the 5-Item Dry Eye Questionnaire (DEQ-5): discrimination across self-assessed severity and aqueous tear deficient dry eye diagnoses. *Cont Lens Anterior Eye.* 2010;33(2):55-60.

17. Nichols KK, Nichols JJ, Mitchell GL. The reliability and validity of McMonnies Dry Eye Index. *Cornea.* 2004;23(4):365-371.

18. Abetz L, Rajagopalan K, Mertzanis P, et al. Development and validation of the Impact of Dry Eye on Everyday Life (IDEEL) questionnaire, a patient-reported outcomes (PRO) measure for the assessment of the burden of dry eye on patients. *Health Qual Life Outcomes.* 2011;9:111.

19. Mangione CM, Lee PP, Gutierrez PR, et al. Development of the 25-item National Eye Institute Visual Function Questionnaire. *Arch Ophthalmol.* 2001;119(7):1050-1058.

20. Revicki DA, Rentz AM, Harnam N, et al. Reliability and validity of the National Eye Institute Visual Function Questionnaire-25 in patients with age-related macular degeneration. *Invest Ophthalmol Vis Sci.* 2010;51(2):712-717.

21. Owen CG, Rudnicka AR, Smeeth L, et al. Is the NEI VFQ-25 a useful tool in identifying visual impairment in an elderly population? *BMC Ophthalmol.* 2006;6:24.

22. Amparo F, Schaumberg DA, Dana R. Comparison of two questionnaires for dry eye symptom assessment: the Ocular Surface Disease Index and the Symptom Assessment in Dry Eye. *Ophthalmology.* 2015;122(7):1498-1503.

23. Qazi Y, Hurwitz S, Khan S, et al. Validity and reliability of a novel Ocular Pain Assessment Survey (OPAS) in quantifying and monitoring corneal and ocular surface pain. *Ophthalmology.* 2016;123(7):1458-1468.

24. Caraceni A, Cherny N, Fainsinger R, et al. Pain measurement tools and methods in clinical research in palliative care: recommendations of an Expert Working Group of the European Association of Palliative Care. *J Pain Symptom Manage.* 2002;23(3):239-255.

25. Farrar JT, Young JP Jr, LaMoreaux L, et al. Clinical importance of changes in chronic pain intensity measured on an 11-point numerical pain rating scale. *Pain.* 2001;94(2):149-158.

26. Paice JA, Cohen FL. Validity of a verbally administered numeric rating scale to measure cancer pain intensity. *Cancer Nurs.* 1997;20(2):88-93.

27. Ferreira-Valente MA, Pais-Ribeiro JL, Jensen MP. Validity of four pain intensity rating scales. *Pain.* 2011;152(10):2399-2404.

28. Jensen MP, Turner JA, Romano JM. What is the maximum number of levels needed in pain intensity measurement? *Pain.* 1994;58(3):387-392.

29. Dworkin RH, Turk DC, Farrar JT, et al. Core outcome measures for chronic pain clinical trials: IMMPACT recommendations. *Pain*. 2005;113(1-2):9-19.

30. Bouhassira D, Attal N, Fermanian J, et al. Development and validation of the Neuropathic Pain Symptom Inventory. *Pain*. 2004;108(3):248-257.

31. Zelman DC, Dukes E, Brandenburg N, et al. Identification of cut-points for mild, moderate and severe pain due to diabetic peripheral neuropathy. *Pain*. 2005;115(1-2):29-36.

32. Spierer O, Felix ER, McClellan AL, et al. Corneal mechanical thresholds negatively associate with dry eye and ocular pain symptoms. *Invest Ophthalmol Vis Sci*. 2016;57(2):617-625.

CHAPTER 4

Does Anyone Do Schirmer Testing Anymore?

Bryan Roth, MD and Elizabeth Yeu, MD

KEY POINTS

- Office diagnostics have evolved to include objective measurements (tear osmolarity, matrix metalloproteinase-9, lactoferrin, Sjögren syndrome testing) and imaging (optical coherence tomography, interferometry, keratography, meibography) to assess the eyelid, tear film, and cornea.
- The 15-second phenol red thread test uses a soft and fine thread, which elicits less reflex tearing when compared to the 5-minute Schirmer test blotting paper strips.
- Currently, there is no gold standard in dry eye diagnostics, but testing options have recently grown.

Dry eye is a common complaint and disease state evaluated in the clinical office and yet the tools to assess it vary widely in both form and function. A multitude of tests aim to assess the different mechanisms of tear production, retention, and make-up. Old mainstays (eg, Schirmer testing) continue to be widely used despite proven difficulty with reproducibility, sensitivity and specificity, and patient discomfort.[1-4] Given the multitude of potential etiologies for dry eye, it is of little surprise that no single test is

Mah FS, Rhee MK, eds.
Dry Eye Disease: A Practical Guide (pp 39-48).
© 2019 Taylor & Francis Group.

considered the gold standard in diagnosis.[1,2,5] Newer technology, such as tear osmolarity measurement, biomarker testing (eg, matrix metalloproteinase-9 [MMP-9], lactoferrin), or tear meniscus optical coherence tomography (OCT), hold the promise of helping to further elucidate the cause of dry eye in specific patients, but also have their own limitations and add additional expense.

We have organized a variety of clinical tests to diagnose dry eye by their intended use. This includes assessment of tear secretion (with both reflex and basic secretion), tear clearance, ocular surface damage, tear film stability, tear volume assessment, and osmolarity assessment. Assessing the severity and cause of dry eye is important not only for symptomatic patients but also in identifying those at risk of dry eye in the preoperative cataract or refractive setting.

CONVENTIONAL TESTING:
TEAR SECRETION AND STABILITY

First described by German ophthalmologist Otto Schirmer in 1903,[6] and still arguably the most commonly used tests in clinical practice, the basic secretion and Schirmer tests are conceptually simple tests that help answer a basic question: Is the eye producing an adequate amount of tears?

Nonstandardized use of these tests including varying measurement cut-offs and procedure variability by practitioner (eg, the blotting of residual fluid from the conjunctival cul-de-sac, degree of topical anesthesia achieved) produces variable results. A multitude of reports illustrate the high variability and poor correlation of these tests with other signs and symptoms of dry eye.[4,7-11] Lucca et al, for example, found Schirmer testing yielded a 25% sensitivity and 90% specificity.[12] Other studies have questioned the repeatability of the tests.[7,13,14] Nichols et al found that simple symptom assessment and tear break-up time (TBUT) were each a more reproducible measure than Schirmer testing, although the authors note that the test performs relatively better with more advanced disease.[4]

Classically, these tests are thought to assess either basal or reflex tearing depending on method and use of a topical anesthetic. Many authors, however, have dismissed the idea that either basal or reflex tearing can be appropriately isolated.[3,15] For example, simple eyelid margin stimulation associated with the blotting paper of Schirmer testing likely also produces significant reflex tearing.[16]

In order to address many of the limitations of the aforementioned Schirmer testing, the phenol red thread test was developed in the 1980s.[17] This test consists of a cotton thread that has been impregnated with pH-sensitive phenol red. Once in contact with the mild alkalinity of tears, the thread changes in color from yellow to red. As the thread is soft and fine compared to Schirmer testing, basic secretion without reflex tearing is thought to be primarily assessed. The test is more comfortable to the patient (causing less reflex tearing) and is quicker to perform (15 seconds vs 5 minutes), allowing for testing in both adult and pediatric populations. Chiang et al compared normal to dry eyes with both Schirmer testing and phenol red testing, concluding that false-positive rates with phenol red were significantly improved from Schirmer (3% vs 18%).[18] Limitations, however, remain numerous, including low reproducibility and poor correlation with other signs and symptoms of dry eye. In clinical practice, use of the phenol red test has been limited largely due to commercial availability of the product. Even the so-called cut-offs for wetting limits are difficult to use for diagnostic purposes given their high variability.[5,19-21]

Saleh et al[19] studied a population of potential cataract patients in preparatory screening for surgery and found that neither Schirmer nor phenol red testing agrees with symptoms; moreover, the 2 tests were found to have no correlation between each other. Additionally, although the tests assess tear production, they do not attempt to assess tear function or composition of the tear film itself.

TBUT is a frequently used test due to its ease as an in-office quick assessment and readily available fluorescein. This test assesses the time interval between a blink and the first appearance of a dry spot overlying the cornea. Tear film instability is reflected by TBUT and is a common finding associated with decreased tear production as well as increased evaporation, such as with dysfunction of the lipid component of the tear film related to meibomian gland disease. Like other tests in the assessment of dry eye, TBUT suffers from low reproducibility[22] and confounding factors that include the amount of fluid given as a part of fluorescein instillation.[4,23]

Assessment of the ocular surface for staining with fluorescein, rose bengal, and lissamine green (all available as solution or impregnated strips) are widely established methods for dry eye diagnosis that are easily performed in the clinical setting. Fluorescein stains epithelial erosions and exposed basement membrane. Rose bengal and lissamine green stain epithelium when a disruption occurs in the protective mucin coating.[24,25] Disadvantages of these modalities include their intrinsic invasiveness that can result in reflex tearing, although lissamine green avoids the burning associated with rose bengal and is less toxic to healthy epithelial cells.[24,25] Several grading schemes, such as the Van Bijsterveld scoring system, which evaluates the cornea by zone and amount of staining, have been developed to monitor and assess corneal grading in a standardized fashion, which is of particular benefit in clinical trials.[26,27] Grading varies widely between practitioners in clinical practice, however.

NEW MODALITIES

Noninvasive methods of dry eye diagnosis, such as corneal topography, tear interferometry, tear evaporimetry, and tear meniscus examination, are now available to assist in diagnosis.[28] Newer testing devices are attempting to overcome some of the inherit limitations of conventional testing, though many have drawbacks of their own.

Optical Coherence Tomography

Anterior segment optical coherence tomography (AS-OCT) is a noninvasive test and, although costly, is available in many practitioners' offices. The device measures tear meniscus, typically inferior, allowing for precise quantitative readings. Savini et al demonstrated that mean tear meniscus height (TMH) was significantly lower (*P* < .0001) in patients with aqueous tear deficiency (0.13 ± 0.07 mm) than in a normal control group (0.25 ± 0.08 mm).[29]

AS-OCT has been reported to be of high potential for the examination and assessment of tear meniscus because of its speed, high resolution, and ability to provide detailed information about the ocular surface noninvasively.[29-31] AS-OCT findings demonstrated good agreement with patient-reported subjective symptoms.[32,33] Demonstrating the multitude of possible clinical applications with the technology, Hwang et al introduced a method of imaging meibomian glands, suggesting that AS-OCT also can be used in meibomian gland disorders.[34] Expected limitations include in-office time, expense, and limited utility in those with conjunctivochalasis and disorders of eyelid margin continuity, among others.

Interferometry

Interferometry, another imaging modality, allows for the rapid evaluation of the tear film in vivo by recording optical interference of the tear film itself, indicative of the presence of a thin lipid layer.[35,36] Prior studies have demonstrated that when the lipid layer is intact, evaporation represents a small loss of water that is compensated for by the lacrimal gland; however, if absent, then the evaporation increases 4-fold leading to symptoms of dry eye.[37] Noting that exacerbation of dry eye syndrome (DES) after phacoemulsification is a common cause of patient dissatisfaction, Kim et al[38] assessed the tear film lipid layer thickness before and after cataract surgery using the LipiView (TearScience), the first device to quantify the tear film lipid layer thickness. The researchers found that the tear film lipid layer was significantly thinner after cataract surgery and that the layer was significantly correlated with DES, suggesting that clinicians should consider the tear film lipid layer while managing the exacerbation of DES after cataract surgery.

Keratography

The OCULUS Keratograph 5M (OCULUS), one of a subset of new advanced corneal topographers, uses infrared light to offer noninvasive keratograph TBUT, TMH, and meibography tools.[39-41] Abdelfattah et al[40] compared this new tool in patients with ocular surface disease to standard controls as well as to more traditional methods (such as fluorescein staining). This group found that OCULUS TMH values were statistically significantly higher in the ocular surface disease group than the control group (0.4:0.3 mm, *P* = .001), whereas traditional fluorescein values were higher in the control group (0.4:0.2 mm, *P* = .01).[40] OCULUS TBUT values were not statistically significantly different between the ocular surface disease and control groups (6.7:8.2 seconds, *P* = .69), whereas fluorescein break-up time values were statistically significantly higher in the control group (6.7:5.6 seconds, *P* = .05). Tian et al found that measurements of TMH and TBUT with this device provide acceptable repeatability and reproducibility, although more so with TMH.[39] Again, this highlights the difficulty in comparing new technology to prior traditional methods in the absence of a gold standard, especially when the prior methods have proven to be poorly reproducible.

Osmolarity

Patients with dry eye have also been shown to have tear film hyperosmolarity. The previously mentioned techniques largely focus on imaging to detail the tear surface; however, the make-up of the tears may hold further diagnostic clues. Previously, difficulties with measuring tear osmolarity have made it cumbersome to measure, but new technologies are quickly altering this. For example, the TearLab Osmolarity System (TearLab), is a hand-held tool that allows for near-instantaneous readings and requires only application to the tear film meniscus for easy measurement. Potvin et al found in a broad study of peer-reviewed literature that the use of tear film osmolarity is supported as an objective numerical measure for diagnosing, grading severity, and managing treatment of dry eye disease.[42] Osmolarity was found to be both repeatable and accurate, and with better sensitivity and specificity than conventional diagnostic techniques.[42-45] Correlations to other forms of testing varied widely, again consistent with the fact that different diagnostic tests reveal different aspects of disease.[46] At present, the consensus cut-off that distinguishes healthy from dry eyes is when the higher tear film osmolarity value of the 2 eyes is 308 mOsm/L,[44,47] or a variance between the eyes, but note that like any diagnostic instrument, interpretation must be based on the entire clinical assessment.[44]

Meibography

Meibomian gland dysfunction (MGD), a common cause of evaporative DES, can be defined as a chronic diffuse abnormality of the meibomian glands caused by either duct obstruction or glandular secretion.[48] Ultimately, these changes lead to altered tear lipid secretions, tear film instability and eventually changes to the ocular surface.[49] Given the importance of MGD as a cause of DES, there are a multitude of new technologies used to assist in its diagnosis. Infrared meibography has previously been used in the clinical setting, enabling 2-dimensional imaging of the meibomian glands to confirm gland dropout[50]; however, detailed anatomic structures cannot be clearly visualized and multiple authors have reported that dropout scores based on infrared images do not correlate with clinical signs, suggesting the need for further methods of evaluation.[51,52]

OCT, previously mentioned for its use in measuring the tear meniscus, is also useful in the diagnosis of MGD. Meibomian gland length and width are noted to be significantly decreased in patients with MGD, and these parameters have been correlated to both ocular surface symptoms and clinical signs.[53] Yoo et al has suggested a discrepancy in the interpretation of 2-dimensional imaging of meibomian glands using infrared meibography as compared to OCT, suggesting that OCT is a more accurate form of diagnosis.[54]

Limitations to this improved imaging exist, and results must be used in the setting of other clinical findings. For example, meibomian gland loss and meibum quality demonstrate a positive correlation to each other but TBUT and corneal staining scores are significantly correlated only with meibum grade, not meibomian gland loss, noting that expression of meibum during slit-lamp examination is still a vital part in diagnosis.[55] This finding by Eom et al[55] illustrates that diagnostics like meibography are helpful, but alone may be insufficient. Furthermore, Kim et al point out that while morphology and function of meibomian glands can be well correlated, a large discrepancy with true function can still exist in hypersecretory MGD or mixed mechanism MGD.[56] Therefore, while meibography is a useful diagnostic assessment tool, it is not specific enough to rule out functional MGD.

Biomarker Assessment

Dry eye is a multifactorial disease requiring a multifactorial approach to diagnosis. One factor that is becoming ever more apparent is the presence or absence of inflammation, the identification of which can help guide therapeutic decision-making.[57] Although there are many inflammatory mediators, MMP-9 serves as an excellent biomarker for inflammation as it elevates early, catalyzes further development of interleukin 1 and tumor necrosis factor-alpha, and accumulates with persistent inflammation.[58-60] Moreover, MMP-9 destabilizes the tear film and directly contributes to corneal barrier dysfunction.[61] Elevation of MMP-9 has been shown to precede the development of corneal staining and contributes to the instability of the tear film in 30% of patients.[62] Interestingly, MMP-9 knockout mice are resistant to developing dry eye.[63]

InflammaDry (Quidel) is a rapid in-office test that simply detects the presence of MMP-9; it does not give a quantitative result. Identifying which symptomatic dry eye patients have underlying inflammation may predict patient responses to treatment and therefore influence clinical management strategy.[64,65] Messmer et al found that MMP-9 results indicated clinically significant inflammation in 40% of dry eye patients, and results correlated well with TBUT, Schirmer testing, conjunctival and corneal staining, number of obstructed meibomian gland ducts, and pathologic meibomian gland secretion.[65]

Lactoferrin, a glycoprotein produced by the lacrimal gland, has also been extensively studied and found to have anti-inflammatory properties.[66] Tear lactoferrin level has been reported as an indicator of lacrimal secretory function. Previous studies reported that tear lactoferrin level correlated with the severity of conjunctivocorneal epithelial lesions in patients with primary, secondary, and non–Sjögren syndrome dry eyes.[67] In practice, the Touch Tear Lactoferrin MicroAssay (Touch Scientific, Inc) and the Tearscan (Advanced Tear Diagnostics) allow for the rapid detection of lactoferrin in tears, with lower levels indicative of dry eye. Oral lactoferrin has been suggested as a treatment modality for improving tear stability and the ocular surface in Sjögren syndrome and may suggest beneficial effects to supplementation.[68]

Sjögren syndrome is an autoimmune disease that often initially presents with nonspecific symptoms including dry eye and dry mouth. Classically, biomarker assessment with SS-A, SS-B, antinuclear antibody, and rheumatoid factor have been used to assist in diagnosis. However, an in-office diagnostic test is now commercially available (Sjö, Bausch + Lomb) that includes novel autoantibodies which appear to be associated with early stages of Sjögren syndrome: salivary protein-1, carbonic anhydrase-6, and parotid secretory protein.[69,70] A blood sample is obtained by an in-office finger prick or collection at a diagnostic laboratory. The test provides greater sensitivity and specificity compared to traditional testing alone as well as the potential for earlier diagnosis.[71-74]

Differentiating between DES and ocular allergy can be a challenge to clinically differentiate. With 30 million Americans affected by seasonal allergies, and 70% of these reporting ocular symptoms, it is important to understand the primary cause of a patient's complaints in order to institute the best treatment.[75] Doctor's Rx Allergy Formula (Bausch + Lomb) is a proprietary in-office diagnostic test that provides allergy testing utilizing a plastic, skin-prick test applicator of 58 allergens. The tests are tailored to be ocular specific and regionalized allowing for the physician to then appropriately manage the primary cause of ocular irritation.

SUMMARY

Dry eye is a frequent problem in the clinical setting, yet the myriad testing available only serves to highlight the difficulty with diagnosing and assessing severity. As outlined previously, each test presents its own challenges to the clinician, whether it is in reliability, sensitivity, or specificity. As dry eye can be a result of poor tear production, retention, or make-up of the tear film itself, no test has proven to effectively diagnose each component individually. Without a reliable gold standard as comparison, even the task of assessing newer modalities has proven challenging. A proficient clinician will seek to use signs and symptomatology of dry eye with ready knowledge of the limitation of each diagnostic tool, whether conventional or newer technology, to best serve their patients.

REFERENCES

1. Smith J, Nichols KK, Baldwin EK. Current patterns in the use of diagnostic tests in dry eye evaluation. *Cornea*. 2008;27:656-662.
2. Versura P, Frigato M, Cellini M, et al. Diagnostic performance of tear function tests in Sjögren's syndrome patients. *Eye*. 2007;21:229-237.
3. Clinch TE, Benedetto DA, Felberg NT, Laibson PR. Schirmer's test. A closer look. *Arch Ophthalmol*. 1983;101:1383-1386.
4. Nichols KK, Mitchell GL, Zadnik K . The repeatability of clinical measurements of dry eye. *Cornea*. 2004;23:272-285.
5. International Dry Eye Workshop. Methodologies to diagnose and monitor dry eye disease: report of the Diagnostic Methodology Subcommittee of the International Dry Eye WorkShop. *Ocul Surf.* 2007;5:108-152.
6. Schirmer O. Studien zur physiologie und pathologie der tranen-absonderung und tranenabfuhr. *Graefes Arch Clin Exp Ophthalmol*. 1903;56:197-291.
7. Cho P, Yap M. Schirmer test II. A clinical study of its repeatability. Optom Vis Sci. 1993;70:157-159.
8. Cho P. Schirmer test I. A review. *Optom Vis Sci*. 1993;70(2):152-156.
9. Kallarackal GU, Ansari EA, Amos N, et al. A comparative study to assess the clinical use of fluorescein meniscus time (FMT) with tear break up time (TBUT) and Schirmer's tests (ST) in the diagnosis of dry eye. *Eye*. 2002;16:594-600.

10. Tomlinson A, Blades KJ, Pearce EI. What does the phenol red thread test actually measure? *Optom Vis Sci.* 2001;78:142-146.

11. Senchyna M, Wax MB. Quantitative assessment of tear production: a review of methods and utility in dry eye drug discovery. *J Ocul Biol Dis Infor.* 2008;1(1):1-6.

12. Lucca JA, Nunez JN, Farris RL. A comparison of diagnostic tests for keratoconjunctivitis sicca: lactoplate, Schirmer, and tear osmolarity. *CLAO J.* 1990;16:109-112.

13. Lee JH, Hyun PM. The reproducibility of the Schirmer test. Korean J Ophthalmol, 1988;2:5-8.

14. Pinschmidt NW. Evaluation of the Schirmer tear test. *South Med J.* 1970;63:1256.

15. Afonso AA, Monroy D, Stern ME, et al. Correlation of tear clearance and Schirmer test scores with ocular irritation symptoms. *Ophthalmology.* 1999;106:803-810.

16. Tabak S. A short Schirmer tear test. *Contacto.* 1972;16:38-42.

17. Hamano HM, Hori M, Hamano T, et al. A new method for measuring tears. *CLAO J.* 1983;9:281-289.

18. Chiang B, Asbell PA, Franklin B. Phenol-red thread test and Schirmer test for tear production in normal and dry eye patients. *Invest Ophthalmol Vis Sci.* 1988;29(Suppl):337.

19. Saleh TA, Bates AK, Ewings P. Phenol red thread test vs Schirmer's test: a comparative study. *Eye.* 2006;20:913-915.

20. Sakamoto R, Bennett ES, Henry VA, et al. The phenol red thread tear test: a cross cultural study. *Invest Ophthalmol Vis Sci.* 1993;34:3510-3514.

21. Cho P. The cotton thread test: a brief review and a clinical study of its reliability on Hong Kong-Chinese. *Optom Vis Sci.* 1993;70:804-808.

22. Vanley GT, Leopold IH, Gregg TH. Interpretation of tear film breakup. *Arch Ophthalmol.* 1977;95:445-448.

23. Johnson ME, Murphy PJ. The effect of instilled fluorescein solution volume on the values and repeatability of TBUT measurements. *Cornea.* 2005;24:811-817.

24. Kim J, Foulks GN. Evaluation of the effect of lissamine green and rose bengal on human corneal epithelial cells. *Cornea.* 1999;18:328-332.

25. Kim J. The use of vital dyes in corneal disease. *Curr Opin Ophthalmol.* 2000;11(4):241-247.

26. Sron AJ, Evans VE, Smith IA. Grading of corneal and conjunctival staining in the context of other dry eye tests. *Cornea.* 2003;22(7):640-650.

27. van Bijsterveld OP. Diagnostic tests in the sicca syndrome. *Arch Ophthalmol.* 1969;82:10-14.

28. Yokoi N, Komuro A. Non-invasive methods of assessing the tear film. *Exp Eye Res.* 2004;78:399-407.

29. Savini G, Barboni P, Zanini M. Tear meniscus evaluation by optical coherence tomography. *Ophthalmic Surg Lasers Imaging.* 2006;37:112-118.

30. Wang J, Aquavella J, Palakuru J, et al. Relationships between central tear film thickness and tear menisci of the upper and lower eyelids. *Invest Ophthalmol Vis Sci.* 2006;47:4349-4355.

31. Ibrahim OM, Dogru M, Takano Y, et al. Application of Visante optical coherence tomography tear meniscus height measurement in the diagnosis of dry eye disease. *Ophthalmology.* 2010;117(10):1923-1929.

32. Nguyen P, Huang D, Li Y, et al. Correlation between optical coherence tomography-derived assessments of lower tear meniscus parameters and clinical features of dry eye disease. *Cornea.* 2012;31(6):680-685.

33. Akiyama R, Usui T, Yamagami S. Diagnosis of dry eye by tear meniscus measurements using anterior segment swept source optical coherence tomography. *Cornea.* 2015;34(Suppl 11):S115-S120.

34. Hwang HS, Shin JG, Lee BH, Eom TJ, Joo C-K. In vivo 3D meibography of the human eyelid using real time imaging fourier-domain OCT. *PLoS ONE.* 2013;8(6).

35. Goto E, Dogru M, Kojima T, Tsubota K. Computer-synthesis of an interference color chart of human tear lipid layer, by a colorimetric approach. *Invest Ophthalmol Vis Sci.* 2003;44(11):4693-4697.

36. Maissa C, Guillon M. Tear film dynamics and lipid layer characteristics: Effect of age and gender. *Cont Lens Anterior Eye.* 2010;33(4):176-182.

37. Mathers WD. Evaporation from the ocular surface. *Exp Eye Res.* 2004;78:389-394.

38. Kim JS, Lee H, Choi S, Kim EK, Seo KY, Kim T. Assessment of the tear film lipid layer thickness after cataract surgery. *Semin Ophthalmol.* 2018;33(2):231-236.

39. Tian L, Qu J, zhang X, Sun X. Repeatability and reproducibility of noninvasive keratograph 5M measurements in patients with dry eye disease. *J Ophthalmol.* 2016;2016:8013621.

40. Abdelfattah NS, Dastiridou A, Sadda SR, Lee OL. Noninvasive imaging of tear film dynamics in eyes with ocular surface disease. *Cornea.* 2015;34(Suppl 10):S48-S52.

41. Khanal S, Tomlinson A, McFadyen A, et al. Dry eye diagnosis. *Invest Ophthalmol Vis Sci.* 2008;49:1407-1414.

42. Potvin R, Makari S, Rapuano CJ. Tear film osmolarity and dry eye disease: a review of the literature. *Clin Ophthalmol (Auckland, NZ).* 2015;9:2039-2047.

43. Versura P, Profazio V, Campos EC. Performance of tear osmolarity compared to previous diagnostic tests for dry eye diseases. *Curr Eye Res.* 2010;35(7):553-564.

44. Lemp MA, Bron AJ, Baudouin C, et al. Tear osmolarity in the diagnosis and management of dry eye disease. *Am J Ophthalmol.* 2011;151(5):792-798.e1.

45. Tomlinson A, Khanal S, Ramaesh K, Diaper C, McFadyen A. Tear film osmolarity: determination of a referent for dry eye diagnosis. *Invest Ophthalmol Vis Sci.* 2006;47(10):4309-4315.

46. Sullivan BD, Crews LA, Messmer EM, et al. Correlations between commonly used objective signs and symptoms for the diagnosis of dry eye disease: clinical implications. *Acta Ophthalmol.* 2014;92(2):161-166.

47. Jacobi C, Jacobi A, Kruse FE, Cursiefen C. Tear film osmolarity measurements in dry eye disease using electrical impedance technology. *Cornea.* 2011;30(12):1289-1292.

48. Nelson JD, Shimazaki J, Benitez-del-Castillo JM, et al. The International Workshop on Meibomian Gland Dysfunction: report of the definition and classification subcommittee. *Invest Ophthalmol Vis Sci.* 2011;52:1930-1937.

49. Knop E, Knop N, Millar T, et al. The International Workshop on Meibomian Gland Dysfunction: report of the subcommittee on anatomy, physiology, and pathophysiology of the meibomian gland. *Invest Ophthalmol Vis Sci.* 2011;52:1938-1978.

50. Arita R, Itoh K, Inoue K, Amano S. Noncontact infrared meibography to document age-related changes of the meibomian glands in a normal population. *Ophthalmology.* 2008;115:911-915.

51. Finis D, Ackermann P, Pischel N, et al. Evaluation of meibomian gland dysfunction and local distribution of meibomian gland atrophy by non-contact infrared meibography. *Curr Eye Res.* 2015;40(10):982-989.

52. Ngo W, Srinivasan S, Schulze M, Jones L. Repeatability of grading meibomian gland dropout using two infrared systems. *Optom Vis Sci.* 2014;91:658-667.

53. Liang Q, Pan Z, Zhou M, et al. Evaluation of optical coherence tomography meibography in patients with obstructive meibomian gland dysfunction. *Cornea.* 2015;34(10):1193-1199.

54. Yoo YS, Na KS, Byun YS, et al. Examination of gland dropout detected on infrared meibography by using optical coherence tomography meibography. *Ocul Surf.* 2017;15(1):130-138.

55. Eom Y, Choi KE, Kang SY, Lee HK, Kim HM, Song JS. Comparison of meibomian gland loss and expressed meibum grade between the upper and lower eyelids in patients with obstructive meibomian gland dysfunction. *Cornea.* 2014;33(5):448-452.

56. Kim HM, Eom Y, Song JS. The relationship between morphology and function of the meibomian glands. *Eye Contact Lens.* 2018;44(1):1-5.

57. Kaufman HE. The practical detection of mmp-9 diagnoses ocular surface disease and may help prevent its complications. *Cornea.* 2013;32(2):211-216.

58. Chotikavanich S, de Paiva CS, Li de Q, et al. Production and activity of matrix metalloproteinase-9 on the ocular surface increase in dysfunctional tear syndrome. *Invest Ophthalmol Vis Sci.* 2009;50(7):3203-3209.

59. Li DQ, Chen Z, Song XJ, Luo L, Pflugfelder SC. Stimulation of matrix metalloproteinases by hyperosmolarity via a JNK pathway in human corneal epithelial cells. *Invest Ophthalmol Vis Sci.* 2004;45(12):4302-4311.

60. Massingale ML, Li X, Vallabhajosyula M, Chen D, Wei Y, Asbell PA. Analysis of inflammatory cytokines in the tears of dry eye patients. *Cornea.* 2009;28(9):1023-1027.

61. Corrales RM, Stern ME, De Paiva CS, Welch J, Li DQ, Pflugfelder SC. Desiccating stress stimulates expression of matrix metalloproteinases by the corneal epithelium. *Invest Ophthalmol Vis Sci.* 2006;47(8):3293-3302.

62. Sambursky R, Davitt WF 3rd, Friedberg M, Tauber S. Prospective, multicenter, clinical evaluation of point-of-care matrix metalloproteinase-9 test for confirming dry eye disease. *Cornea.* 2014;33(8):812-818.

63. Pflugfelder SC, de Paiva CS, Tong L, Luo L, Stern ME, Li DQ. Stress-activated protein kinase signaling pathways in dry eye and ocular surface disease. *Ocul Surf.* 2005;3(Suppl 4):S154-S157.

64. Sambursky R. Presence or absence of ocular surface inflammation directs clinical and therapeutic management of dry eye. *Clin Ophthalmol (Auckland, NZ)*. 2016;10:2337-2343.

65. Messmer EM, von Lindenfels V, Garbe A, Kampik A. Matrix metalloproteinase 9 testing in dry eye disease using a commercially available point-of-care immunoassay. *Ophthalmology*. 2016;123(11):2300-2308.

66. Conneely OM. Antiinflammatory activities of lactoferrin. *J Am Coll Nutr*. 2001;20(5 Suppl):389S-395S.

67. Danjo Y, Lee M, Horimoto K, Hamano T. Ocular surface damage and tear lactoferrin in dry eye syndrome. *Acta Ophthalmol (Copenh)*. 1994;72:433-437.

68. Dogru M, Matsumoto Y, Yamamoto Y, et al. Lactoferrin in Sjogren's syndrome. *Ophthalmology*. 2007;114(12):2366-2367.

69. Shen L, Suresh L, Lindemann M, et al. Novel autoantibodies in Sjogren's syndrome. *Clin Immunol*. 2012;145:251-255.

70. Shen L, Kapsoqeorqou EK, Yu M, et al. Evaluation of salivary gland protein 1 antibodies in patients with primary and secondary Sjogren's syndrome. *Clin Immunol*. 2014;155:42-46.

71. Matossian C, Micucci J. Characterization of the serological biomarkers associated with Sjogren's syndrome in patients with recalcitrant dry eye disease. *Clin Ophthalmol*. 2016;10:1329-1334.

72. Beckman KA, Luchs J, Milner MS. Making the diagnosis of Sjogren's syndrome in patients with dry eye. *Clin Ophthalmol*. 2016;10:43-53.

73. Suresh L, Malyavantham K, Shen L, Ambrus JL, Jr. Investigation of novel autoantibodies in Sjögren's syndrome utilizing Sera from the Sjögren's international collaborative clinical alliance cohort. *BMC Ophthalmol*. 2015;15(1):38.

74. Beckman KA. Detection of early markers for Sjögren syndrome in dry eye patients. *Cornea*. 2014;33(12):1262-1264.

75. Singh K, Axelrod S, Bielory L. The epidemiology of ocular and nasal allergy in the United States, 1988-1994. *J Allergy Clin Immunol*. 2010;126(4):778-783.e6.

CHAPTER 5

What About the Eyelids?

Katherine Duncan, MD and Jenny Y. Yu, MD, FACS

KEY POINTS

- Abnormal eyelid position and function are overlooked contributors to dry eye disease.
- Dry eye is reported in up to 25% of patients after blepharoplasty.
- Facial nerve palsy affects blinking and closure of the eye, resulting in corneal exposure.
- Eyelid pathology can be effectively addressed by medical and/or surgical options to improve dry eye.

Eyelid structure, position, and function are often-overlooked contributors to dry eye disease (DED). The function of the eyelids is to protect the surface of the eye and facilitate distribution of the tear film. Their anatomical structure and position can often exacerbate DED. This chapter will review the most common pathologic and age-related changes of the eyelids that result in dry eye.

Mah FS, Rhee MK, eds.
Dry Eye Disease: A Practical Guide (pp 48-56).
© 2019 Taylor & Francis Group.

ANATOMY/FUNCTION

A detailed understanding of the normal eyelid anatomy is crucial to properly identifying any eyelid pathology that may be contributing to dry eye. The upper and lower
eyelids surround the palpebral fissure. The structure of the palpebral fissure is maintained by the medial and lateral canthal tendons. The lateral canthal tendon attaches
2 mm above the medial canthal tendon. The medial canthal tendon splits around the
lacrimal sac before attaching to the lacrimal crests. With the eye in primary position,
the margin of the upper eyelid should cover the superior 1 to 2 mm of the cornea, while
the margin of the lower eyelid is usually within 2 mm of the inferior border of the cornea. The main retractor of the upper eyelids is the levator muscle, innervated by cranial
nerve III. The main protractor of the eyelids is the orbicularis oculi muscle, innervated
by cranial nerve VII. The layers of the eyelid can be divided into the anterior (skin,
orbicularis) and posterior (tarsus and conjunctiva) lamellae. The eyelid margin serves
as the junction of the conjunctiva, orbicularis, and cutaneous epithelium. The tear film
is composed of oil, mucin, and aqueous. The eyelid margins are lined by oil-secreting
meibomian glands. The conjunctiva contains mucin-secreting goblet cells as well as
aqueous-secreting accessory lacrimal glands. The main lacrimal gland sits in the superolateral orbit and secretes aqueous into the superolateral fornix. Pathology affecting any
of these structures has the potential to exacerbate dry eye.[1,2]

AGE-RELATED CHANGES

Loss of skin elasticity, soft tissue atrophy, skeletal remodeling, and sun exposure contribute to the changes that occur in the periocular region with age. More specifically,
canthal tendon laxity and atrophy of the tarsus result in increased horizontal laxity of
the eyelids. Horizontal laxity decreases the stability of the eyelids and increases the risk
of entropion or ectropion (Figure 5-1).[3] The conjunctival surface of the inner eyelid,
termed the *lid wiper*, is composed of thickened epithelium and goblet cells. This area of
the inner eyelid is specifically designed to maintain tight contact with the bulbar surface
of the globe, allowing it to act as a specialized lubrication system for evenly coating the
ocular surface with tear film during a blink.[4] As the eyelids become increasingly lax
with age, their ability to function properly in distributing the tear film becomes compromised. Patients with eyelid laxity are known to have more dry eye symptoms, decreased
tear break-up times, increased corneal staining, and decreased Schirmer test scores.[5]

Evaluating the eyelids for age-related laxity begins with checking the position of the
eyelid margin. The eyelid margins should be well apposed to the globe with the lower
eyelid margin sitting within 2 mm of the inferior limbus. Inward or outward rotation
of the eyelid margin indicates entropion/ectropion, which is most often a result of
eyelid laxity. Pulling the lower eyelid downward, away from the globe, and evaluating
how quickly it returns to its normal position is known as a *snap back* test. A delayed
or incomplete snap back is indicative of eyelid laxity. The ability to excessively distract
the lower eyelid from the globe surface is another indicator for laxity. Eyelid laxity can

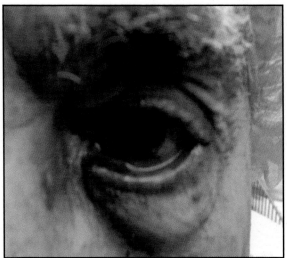

Figure 5-1. Ectropion of the lower eyelid due to laxity.

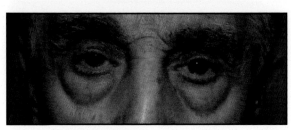

Figure 5-2. Festooning of the lower eyelid fat pads.

be addressed relatively easily with a eyelid tightening procedure, such as a lateral tarsal strip or a wedge resection. Festooning of the lower eyelid fat pads can also contribute to mild ectropion (Figure 5-2). This should be taken into consideration when assessing the patient. Eyelid retraction with mid-face descent can often contribute to dry eye as well (Figure 5-3). It is often overlooked as subtle vertical displacement and/or rounding of the lower eyelids lateral to the lateral limbus. The vertical displacement rather than horizontal laxity increases the ocular surface to more exposure, exacerbating dry eye symptoms. Treatment for aging-related eyelid retraction can include lengthening the lower eyelids with a spacer and/or a mid-face lift through a lateral canthal approach.

CICATRICIAL CHANGES

Cicatricial eyelid changes can be caused by various skin conditions, trauma, and surgical complications. These changes have the potential to interfere with the normal position and function of the eyelids. Blepharoplasty is one of the most commonly preformed procedures in the United States by surgeons of many different specialties. Preoperative evaluation should include a baseline assessment for signs and symptoms of dry eye. However, many surgeons performing these operations do not have the equipment or

Figure 5-3. Eyelid retraction with mid-face descent.

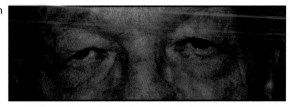

Figure 5-4. Cicatricial eyelid retraction after orbital fracture repair.

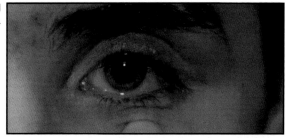

Figure 5-5. Cicatricial lagophthalmos after an eyelid laceration.

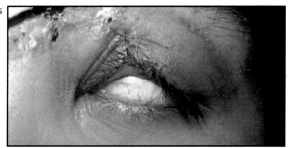

training to thoroughly evaluate for the condition. Upper and lower eyelid blepharoplasties typically involve the removal of skin and occasionally orbicularis from the eyelids. Removing too much tissue can result in postoperative lagophthalmos and ectropion. The transconjunctival approach for a lower eyelid blepharoplasty may result in scarring and shortening of the posterior lamella and therefore has the potential to result in entropion. Dry eye is reported in up to 25% of patients after blepharoplasty and often goes on to become a chronic condition.[6]

Orbital floor fracture repair is approached either transconjunctivally or with an external subciliary incision in the lower eyelid. In either case, a common complication of this procedure is cicatricial lower eyelid retraction, occurring much more frequently with the external subciliary approach (Figure 5-4).[7] The lower eyelid retraction in this instance can result in exposure and chronic inflammation and can be very debilitating.

Lacerations, burns, infections, and dermatologic disorders can also result in scarring of the eyelid tissue, distorting its normal architecture and position (Figure 5-5). Scarring to any layer of the eyelids can also result in the function of the eyelids decreasing the distribution of the tear film.

Patients with dry eyes should be asked pertinent history of eyelid surgery, trauma, or dermatologic conditions. Position and closure of the eyelids should be assessed. Cicatricial changes that result in eyelid malposition are often addressed with surgical release of scar tissue as well as skin or mucosal grafting.

NEUROLOGIC PATHOLOGY AFFECTING EYELID FUNCTION

Eyelid position and function is highly dependent on the normal neurologic innervation of the eyelid musculature. Any disruption to the ability of the orbicularis muscle to function in blinking and closure of the eye can result in dry eye and corneal exposure. This is most clearly exemplified in patients with facial nerve palsy. Facial nerve palsy can be infectious, inflammatory, neoplastic, traumatic, or idiopathic in etiology. The House-Brackmann grading scale can be used to assess dynamic facial nerve function in these cases.[8] Patients with facial nerve palsy develop widening of the palpebral fissure, loss of the blink reflex, reduced tear production, paralytic ectropion of the lower eyelids, and lagophthalmos. They all contribute to dry eye. Management of these patients is best undertaken in a staged fashion depending on the severity and prognosis of the palsy. Lubrication, tarsorrhaphy, upper eyelid loading procedures, lower eyelid ectropion repair, brow ptosis repair, and mid-face lift are options for management.[9]

Though there are various surgical options for correcting position and closure, the blink rate often remains reduced, affecting the distribution of the tear film.

Although facial dystonias are not considered a cause of dry eye, they are often associated with dry eye and therefore should be considered when assessing patients with dry eye symptoms. Benign essential blepharospasm is a condition characterized by frequent blinking and involuntary spasm of the eyelid protractors (Figure 5-6). The majority of patients who develop blepharospasm suffer from dry eye prior to developing the dystonia.[10] Hemifacial spasm is characterized by episodic contracture of one side of the face. It is often seen in patients with facial nerve weakness and can be the result of vascular compression of the facial nerve or aberrant regeneration after facial nerve palsy. Both conditions can be associated with dry eye, can be functionally debilitating, and are best treated with neurotoxin injections.[11]

SYSTEMIC CONDITIONS AFFECTING EYELID FUNCTION

Thyroid eye disease and floppy eyelid syndrome represent periocular manifestations of systemic diseases that adversely affect eyelid function and can contribute to dry eye. Thyroid eye disease develops in half of patients with systemic thyroid disease. The pathophysiology is poorly understood, but it is felt that autoantibodies against thyroid receptors cross-react with orbital antigens and produce an inflammatory response

Figure 5-6. Eyelid spasm characteristic of blepharospasm.

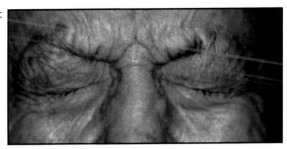

Figure 5-7. Lower eyelid retraction and proptosis characteristic of thyroid eye disease.

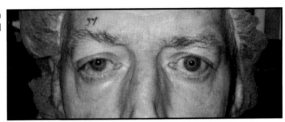

resulting in edema, fibrosis, and adipogenesis within the orbit. These changes manifest clinically as eyelid retraction, proptosis, lagophthalmos, and restrictive strabismus (Figure 5-7). A compressive optic neuropathy is a severe sequela. Dry eye is present in the majority of patients diagnosed with thyroid eye disease and often significantly reduces their quality of life. The mechanism of dry eye in these patients is due to both exposure from their eyelid retraction, proptosis, lagophthalmos, and incomplete blink as well as reduced aqueous tear production due to inflammation.[12] Treatment of dry eye in these patients depends on the activity and severity of their disease. Medical therapy can include lubrication of the ocular surface and closure of the puncta for symptomatic relief as a first line. During the active phase, temporizing measures of improving exposure can also include neurotoxin injections to improve upper eyelid retraction and suture tarsorrhaphy. Systemic steroid is preferred in controlling the active inflammation of the disease. Once the disease is inactive, surgical interventions such as orbital decompression and correction of eyelid malposition are performed if needed to improve exposure and dry eye symptoms.

Floppy eyelid syndrome is a disorder characterized by severe upper eyelid laxity, a soft foldable tarsus, and chronic papillary conjunctivitis. These changes result in upper eyelids that are easily malpositioned and everted, interfering with the eyelid's function to protecting the globe and distribute the tear film. Chronic inflammation caused by eyelid malposition contributes to meibomian gland dysfunction and an unstable tear film composition.[13] Although the exact pathophysiology is unknown, this syndrome is strongly associated with obstructive sleep apnea.[14] Treatment of the patient's sleep apnea with continuous positive airway pressure (CPAP) has been shown to improve floppy eyelid syndrome.[15] Other management strategies include lubrication and tightening procedures, such as a lateral tarsal strip or wedge resection of the upper eyelids.

Cosmetics

Because the eyes are the aesthetic center of the face, an abundance of cosmetics and beauty products are designed to be used on the eyelids. Heavy makeup use can be associated with meibomian gland dysfunction, and patients with dry eye symptoms related to tear film instability should be counseled against this. Latisse (bimatoprost 0.03%) is a commercial product designed to result in longer, thicker eyelashes. Conjunctival hyperemia, pruritis, and punctate keratitis have been reported as adverse effects of Latisse use.[16] Eyelash extension procedures have gained popularity in recent years. These procedures involve securing synthetic eyelashes to the natural eyelash with adhesive glue. This glue has been reported to cause allergic blepharitis and keratoconjunctivitis in some patients and likely also contributes to meibomian gland dysfunction and tear film instability.[17] Eyeliner and makeup tattooing can also affect the health of the meibomian glands, resulting in the dysfunction of the lipid layer of the tear film.

Nonsurgical procedures in the periocular region for rejuvenation continue to grow at a substantial pace. Chemical and laser skin resurfacing can temporarily exacerbate dry eye symptoms. Neurotoxin and collagen filler injections can also contribute to dry eye symptoms when complications affect the blink and closure function of the eyelids. Fat transfers around the periocular region can create ocular surface inflammation and may lead to dry eye symptoms as well. It is important to have a proper history pertaining to the use of these nonsurgical treatments in evaluating a patient with either new and/or worsening dry eye symptoms.

Summary

The eyelids play an integral role in the maintenance of the ocular surface. Any disruption to the normal structure and function of the eyelids has the potential to result in DED. Understanding and identifying pathology of the eyelids is crucial to performing a thorough evaluation of the causes and contributors to dry eye. Eyelid pathology can often be effectively addressed medically and/or surgically to make a substantial improvement in dry eye symptoms.

References

1. Nerad JA. *Techniques in Ophthalmic Plastic Surgery: A Personal tutorial.* London, England: Elsevier; 2010.
2. Holds JB. 2013-2014 Basic and Clinical Science Course: Orbit, Eyelids and Lacrimal System. San Francisco, CA: American Academy of Ophthalmology; 2013.
3. Ko AC, Korn BS, Kikkawa DO. The aging face. *Surv Ophthalmol.* 2017;62(2):190-202. doi:10.1016/j.survophthal.2016.09.002.
4. Knop N, Korb DR, Blackie CA, Knop E. The lid wiper contains goblet cells and goblet cell crypts for ocular surface lubrication during the blink. *Cornea.* 2012;31(3):668-679.
5. Chhadva, P, McClellan AL, Alabiad CR, Feuer WJ, Batawi H, Galor A. Impact of eyelid laxity on symptoms and signs of dry eye disease. *Cornea.* 2016;35:531-535.

6. Prischmann J, Sufyan A, Ting JY, Ruffin C, Perkins SW. Dry eye symptoms and chemosis following blepharoplasty. *JAMA Facial Plast Surg.* 2013;15(1):39-46.
7. Rasche G, Djedovic G, Peisker A, et al. The isolated orbital floor fracture from a transconjunctival or subciliary perspective-A standardized anthropometric evaluation. *Med Oral Patol Oral Cir Bucal.* 2016;21(1):e111-e117.
8. House JW, Brackmann DE. Facial nerve grading system. *Otolaryngol Head Neck Surg.* 1985;93(2):146-147.
9. Rahman I, Sadiq SA. Ophthalmic management of facial nerve palsy: a review. *Surv Ophthalmol.* 2007;52(2):121-144.
10. Lu R, Huang R, Li K, et al. The influence of benign essential blepharospasm on dry eye disease and ocular inflammation. *Am J Ophthalmol.* 2014;157:591-597.
11. Abahneh OH Cetinkaya A, Kulwin DR. Long-term efficacy and safety of botulinum toxin A injections to treat blepharospasm and hemifacial spasm. *Clin Exp Ophthalmol.* 2014;42(3):254-261.
12. Selter JH, Gire AI, Sikder S. The relationship between Graves' ophthalmopathy and dry eye syndrome. *Clin Ophthalmol.* 2015;9:57-62.
13. Liu DT, Di Pascuale MA, Sawai J, Gao Y, Tseng SCG. Tear film dynamics in floppy eyelid syndrome. *Invest Ophthalmol Vis Sci.* 2003;44:1897-1905.
14. Muniesa MJ, Huerva V, Sanchez-de-la-Torre M, Martinez M, Jurjo C, Barbe F. The relationship between floppy eyelid syndrome and obstructive sleep apnea. *Br J Ophthalmol.* 2013;97:1387-1390.
15. McNab AA. Reversal of floppy eyelid syndrome with treatment of obstructive sleep apnoea. *Clin Experiment Ophthalmol.* 2000;28(2):125-126.
16. Ahluwalia GS. Safety and efficacy profile of bimatoprost solution 0.03% topical application in patients with chemotherapy-induced eyelash loss. *J Investig Dermatol Symp Proc.* 2013;16:S73-S76. doi:10.1038/jidsymp.2013.30.
17. Amano Y, Sugimoto Y, Sugita M. Ocular disorders due to eyelash extensions. *Cornea.* 2012;31(2):121-125.

SECTION III

MANAGEMENT OF CASE STUDIES AND CLINICAL SCENARIOS
WHAT IS YOUR APPROACH?

CHAPTER 6

A 25-Year-Old App Designer Who Wears Contacts and Eyelash Extensions

Emily J. Jacobs, MD and Michelle K. Rhee, MD

KEY POINTS

- The average American spends 7 hours per day staring at a screen, an activity which contributes to dry eye. Blink frequency is reduced by 66%, leading to increased evaporation of tears. Positioning the screen 4 to 5 inches below eye level can reduce surface exposure and evaporation.
- Eyelash extensions and eyelid tattooing are popular beauty trends that can be associated with keratoconjunctivitis and tear film instability.
- Patients need to be educated on the dangers of eye whitening, extraocular implants (jewelry inserted beneath the conjunctiva), and unregulated decorative contact lenses.

Today, more than ever, society is dependent on technology. Whether it be a smart phone, tablet, or laptop, the average working American spends multiple hours per day staring at a screen. Computer vision syndrome is not uncommon, and long amounts of screen time can affect the ocular surface and exacerbate the signs and symptoms of dry eye. For many, a portion of daily screen time is dedicated to social media, which often

Mah FS, Rhee MK, eds.
Dry Eye Disease: A Practical Guide (pp 59-66).
© 2019 Taylor & Francis Group.

focuses on beauty trends. Ocular embellishments, such as eyelash extensions, permanent tattoos, eye whitening, and cosmetic eyelid surgery, are often displayed, all of which can cause dry eye disease. Additionally, whether for cosmetic or medical purposes, the use of contact lenses is becoming increasingly popular. When faced with a patient such as the one in the chapter title, education regarding proper contact lens care and the risks of ocular embellishments is critical in the prevention of ocular surface disease.

COMPUTER VISION SYNDROME

Much like the 25-year-old app designer, the average American spends 7 hours per day staring at a screen, and many, up to 72% in one study, experience dry eye symptoms.[1] Symptoms tend to be greater in women and when greater than 6 hours per day is spent on the computer. One study found a significantly lower tear meniscus height in those who wore contact lenses and spent more than 4 hours per day on a computer.[2] On average, blink frequency is reduced 66% while working at a computer. This leads to an increase in the evaporation of tears. A recent study showed decreased concentrations of Mucin 5AC, a lubricant in human tears secreted by goblet cells, in people who use computers for multiple hours per day.[3] The longer the screen time, the less Mucin 5AC was found in tears. Additionally, prolonged screen time can lead to a decrease in tear secretion from the lacrimal gland.[4] Ideally, the screen should be located 4 to 5 inches below eye level to reduce surface exposure and evaporative dry eye symptoms.

EYELASH EXTENSIONS

As demonstrated by our patient, one of the most popular ocular beauty trends is the use of eyelash extensions, which are applied to one's natural eyelashes often using an adhesive agent. The bonding agents commonly contain latex, formaldehyde, or other chemicals, which can damage the ocular surface. In one study of 107 patients without prior eye disease, 64 developed keratoconjunctivitis and 42 developed allergic conjunctivitis, likely due to the glue used during application. Conjunctival erosion as well as subconjunctival hemorrhage were also observed.[5] Another study found that 26.8% of women experienced ocular hyperemia, pain, and itchiness.[6] Wind tunnel experiments have been used to confirm that unnaturally long eyelashes channel airflow and dust particles toward the ocular surface.[7] This escalates shear stress on the ocular surface as well as evaporative dry eye. Additionally, this increase in stress and foreign particles on the dry ocular surface might lead to a higher risk of developing infection.

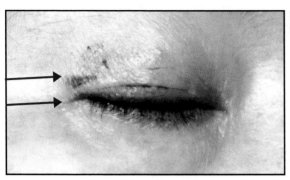

Figure 6-1. (Top arrow) Makeup. (Bottom arrow) Eyeliner tattoo.

EYELID TATTOOING

Many women are now choosing permanent eyeliner in place of the daily application of makeup (Figure 6-1). It has been found that eyelid tattooing decreases tear film stability through the loss of meibomian glands. This, in turn, leads to decreased tear break-up time and an increase in fluorescein staining and corneal erosion.[8] The combination of these effects exacerbates the signs and symptoms of dry eye. A case report shows that even years after eyelid tattooing, a patient presented with decreased tear film stability, increased surface staining, and total meibomian gland dropout bilaterally.[9] Dry eye can also be made worse by disruption of eyelid architecture, as well as by chronic inflammation caused by pigment granules.[10]

EYE WHITENING

Developed in eastern Asia, eye-whitening procedures have been used to treat chronically hyperemic or pigmented eyes. A few techniques have been employed to achieve eye whitening. One of the most common techniques involves extensive conjunctival resection and tenonectomy with topical mitomycin C (MMC) or bevacizumab injections.[11] The I-Brite (Boxer Wachler Vision Institute) eye-whitening system, which also involves conjunctivectomy and MMC, is one option that is available in the United States. There is also an approach that involves the injection of white tattoo ink into the subconjunctival space to achieve a white appearance.[12]

Many studies have shown that complications can arise from these procedures, in as high as over 90% of patients. One study found that 16 out of 17 eyes had persistent conjunctival epithelial defects, with 10 eyes requiring amniotic membrane grafting to facilitate re-epithelialization.[13] In another study of 1713 patients, dry eye was the second most common complication, following fibroproliferation, affecting 32% of patients.[11] The results of a follow-up telephone survey conducted at a mean of 12.9 months after surgery revealed that 56.9% of patients with dry eye symptoms had not experienced an improvement in symptoms or were not satisfied with the results of their surgery.[11] This reflects the critical role that the conjunctiva plays in tear film function. This is supported by another study, which found that 23% of patients suffered from chronic dysfunctional tear syndrome.[14] Limbal stem cell compromise has also been reported.[13] Given the high incidence and severity of complications, including delayed-onset of scleral thinning, patients should be counseled against having this procedure.[15]

BLEPHAROPLASTY

Eyelid surgery, whether done for cosmetic reasons or for visually significant dermatochalasis, can exacerbate dry eye due to an increase in surface exposure. While it should not be relied upon as the sole method of screening dry eye patients, preoperative Schirmer testing has been recommended to identify patients with decreased tear production prior to blepharoplasty.[16] In a survey of 544 oculoplastic surgeons, it was found that 36% perform no tear production tests, 33% perform a test if indicated by signs or symptoms, and only 29% always perform a test.[16] It has been repeatedly shown that both tear quantity and quality can decrease following surgery.[17] In a large 10-year retrospective review of 892 blepharoplasty cases, dry eye symptoms and chemosis were reported in 26.5% and 26.3% of patients, respectively. The same study showed that the incidences of dry eye symptoms and chemosis were significantly higher in patients who underwent concurrent upper and lower blepharoplasty, as well as in patients who experienced postoperative lagophthalmos.[18] Limited skin excision as well as preoperative punctal occlusion has been recommended by some authors to prevent dry eye.[19,20] Despite punctal occlusion, however, some patients still have worsening of dry eye symptoms. Though the exacerbation of dry eye symptoms can be transient, patients should be educated about the side effects of increased ocular surface exposure prior to surgery.

EXTRAOCULAR IMPLANTS

Originally developed at the Netherlands Institute for Innovative Ocular Surgery and coined under the name JewelEye, extraocular implants are now becoming more popular in the United States. This procedure involves the implantation of a small piece of decorative jewelry, generally about 3 mm in size, beneath the superficial layers of the interpalpebral conjunctiva. In 2004, the American Academy of Ophthalmology spoke out against cosmetic implants, stating that they could cause scar tissue, infection, and scleral erosion. Additionally, given the mobility of the conjunctiva, the implant could move causing bleeding and inflammation. This risk of surface inflammation and scarring could increase dry eye symptoms and signs. Patients should be advised against the insertion of extraocular implants.

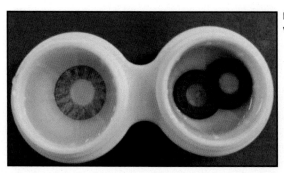

Figure 6-2. Decorative contact lenses without a doctor's prescription.

CONTACT LENSES

Whether for cosmetic or functional purposes, contact lens use is extremely popular, but can have a negative impact on the ocular surface. The International Dry Eye WorkShop report from 2007 found that 50% of contact lens users reported dry eye symptoms.[21] Women were 50% more likely to report symptoms than men. Research has shown that contact lenses decrease tear film thickness and alter the normal tear film dynamics, as the tear film is divided into pre- and post-lens films.[22] Additionally, contact lens wear decreases the stability of the tear film lipid layer due to changes in meibomian gland morphology.[23] In fact, the longer the duration of contact lens wear, the bigger the decrease in number of functional meibomian glands on the eyelids.[24] This, in turn, leads to greater evaporation of the tear film and quicker tear break-up time. Contact lenses with higher water content, in particular, were more vulnerable to drying. Additionally, these contact lenses resulted in thinner tear films with shorter noninvasive break-up. It has been suggested that a pre-lens tear thinning time of less than 3 seconds indicates tear film dysfunction due to contact lens wear.[25]

Research has shown improvement of symptoms in patients who switch to daily disposable contacts.[26] Improvement has also been seen in patients using contact lenses with lower water content and in those who switched to silicone hydrogel contact lenses.[27,28] Switching from multipurpose cleaners to peroxide-based solutions might also help to improve dry eye symptoms.[29] However, this system is not recommended for patients who use contact lenses intermittently, as the contact lenses sit for many days in neutralized solution. The use of artificial tears and punctal plugs has also been recommended. Additionally, omega-3 and omega-6 fatty acid supplements can decrease evaporative tear loss.[30] Patient education and increasing patient compliance regarding contact lens care is of critical importance. Among a general contact lens population, one study found that half of asymptomatic patients during a routine visit presented with signs of treatable contact lens-related complications.[31]

Decorative or cosmetic contact lenses, in particular, can cause significant damage to the ocular surface due to their often unregulated and unsupervised use (Figure 6-2). In collaboration with US Immigration and Customs Enforcement and Homeland Security, the US Federal Drug Administration seized more than 20,000 pairs of illegally imported counterfeit contact lenses in 2013. The following year, 12 defendants in Los Angeles,

Figure 6-3. *Streptococcus keratitis* with hypopyon in decorative contact lens wearer.

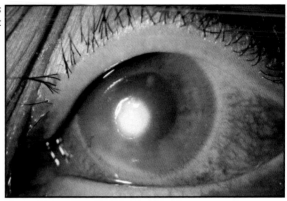

California, were caught selling misbranded and contaminated decorative contact lenses in Halloween stores without doctor's prescriptions. Sale of contact lenses without a doctor's prescription has been illegal in the United States since 2005, as all contact lenses (including plano contact lenses) are deemed medical devices.[32] Despite this legislation, global internet sites provide a loophole that allows for easy purchase of contact lenses without a prescription.

Consumers often purchase these contact lenses without a prescription to change eye color or pupil shape as a beauty trend and for Halloween or other costume play; they are under the erroneous impression that, because there is no refractive prescription to the contact lens, one size fits all and there is no need for an eye exam. Circle contact lenses, which extend well beyond the limbus onto the conjunctiva, can cause damage to the ocular surface due to improper fit. Most worrisome is that the relative risk of developing microbial keratitis in decorative contact lens wearers is increased 16.5 times when compared to the use of prescription contact lenses (Figure 6-3).[33] Young et al reviewed 23 articles of 70 patient cases of unregulated contact lens use. The found that 94% of complications with unregulated contact lenses involved decorative plano contact lenses, 70% of patients had microbial keratitis, and 77% had infection with loss of 2 or more lines of vision.[34]

One study looked at the surface and colorants used in 5 cosmetic contact lenses commercially available in Japan.[35] The study found that the colorants used in the contact lenses contained titanium, iron, and chlorine, which can be toxic to the ocular surface. In another study, 15 brands of decorative contact lenses were evaluated with a rub-off test where a cotton-tip was used to simulate typical contact lens cleaning; only 2 brands did not have pigment rub-off. Furthermore, the colored version of a contact lens where pigment rubbed off had enhanced bacterial adhesion of *Pseudomonas*, *Staphylococcus aureus*, and *Serratia marcescens*, when compared to the same brand's clear contact lens version.[36]

SUMMARY

In a world so largely influenced by technology and social media, society is spending more time than ever on electronic devices and putting ever more emphasis on ocular beauty trends. In addition, access to unregulated products such as decorative contact lenses is easier than ever through the global internet market. Patients need to be educated on the risks of cosmetic products and procedures and the detrimental effects that they can have on the ocular surface. Physicians can report all contact lens infection to the US Federal Drug Administration website MedWatch, as well as report illegal sales to the Federal Trade Commission.

REFERENCES

1. Porcar E, Pons AM, Lorente A. Visual and ocular effects from the use of flat-panel displays. *Int J Ophthalmol.* 2016;9(6):881-885.
2. Kojima T, Ibrahim OM, Wakamatsu T,et al. The impact of contact lens wear and visual display terminal work on ocular surface and tear functions in office workers. *Am J Ophthalmol.* 2011;152(6):933-940.
3. Uchino Y, Uchino M, Yokoi N, et al. Alteration of tear mucin 5AC in office workers using visual display terminals the Osaka study. *JAMA Ophthalmol.* 2014;132(8):985-992.
4. Nakamura S, Kinoshita S, Yokoi N, et al. Lacrimal hypofunction as a new mechanism of dry eye in visual display terminal users. *PLoS One.* 2010;5(6):e11119.
5. Amano Y, Sugimoto Y, Sugita, M. Ocular disorders due to eyelash extensions. *Cornea.* 2012;31:121-125.
6. Amano Y, Nishiwaki Y. National survey on eyelash extensions and their related health problems. *Nihon Eiseigaku Zasshi.* 2013;68(3):168-174.
7. Amador G, Mao W, DeMercurio P, et al. Eyelashes divert airflow to protect the eye. *J R Soc Interface.* 2015;12(105):20141294.
8. Lee Y, Kim J, Hyon J, Wee W, Shin Y. Eyelid tattooing induces meibomian gland loss and tear film instability. *Cornea.* 2015;34:750-755.
9. Kojima T, Dogru M, Matsumoto Y, Goto E, Tsubota K. Tear film and ocular surface abnormalities after eyelid tattooing. *Ophthal Plast Reconstr Surg.* 2005;21:69-71.
10. Morrison CJ, Stam JM. My tattoos caused my dry eye? A new way to look at diagnosis and treatment of patients with tattoo eyeliner. *Canadian Journal of Optometry.* 2016;78(2):6-10.
11. Lee S, Go J, Rhiu S, Stulting RD, et al. Cosmetic regional conjunctivectomy with postoperative mitomycin C application with or without bevacizumab injection. *Am J Ophthalmol.* 2013;156:616-622.
12. Motassian C, Donaldson K, Epitropoulos A, McDonald M. OSD in women, beauty has a price. False lashes, permanent eye makeup, tattoos can cause dry eye. Maybe Keats was referring to natural beauty. *Ophthalmology Management.* 2016;20(4):30-33.
13. Vo RC, Stafeeva K, Aldave AJ, et al. Complications related to a cosmetic eye-whitening procedure. *Am J Ophthalmol.* 2014;158:967-973.
14. Rhiu S, Shim J, Kim EK, Chung SK, Lee JS, Seo KY. Complications of cosmetic wide conjunctivectomy combined with post-surgical mitomycin C to treat chronic hyperemic conjunctiva. *Cornea.* 2012;31:245-252.
15. Saldanha MJ, Yang PT, Chan CC. Scleral thinning after I-BRITE procedure treated with amniotic membrane graft. *Can J Ophthalmol.* 2016;51:e115-116.
16. Esinoza GM, Israel H, Holds JB. Survey of oculoplastic surgeons regarding clinical use of tear production tests. *Ophthalmol Plast Reconstr Surg.* 2009;25(3):197-200.
17. Daily RA, Saulny SM, Sullivan SA, et al. Muller muscle-conjunctival resection: effect on tear production. *Ophthalmol Plast Reconstr Surg.* 2002;18(6):421-425.

18. Prischmann J, Sufyan A, Ting JY, et al. Dry eye symptoms and chemosis following blepharoplasty: a 10-year retrospective review of 892 cases in a single-surgeon series. *JAMA Facial Plast Surg.* 2013;15(1):39-46.

19. Rees TD, Jelks GW. Blepharoplasty and the dry eye syndrome: guidelines for surgery. *Plast Reconstr Surg.* 1981;68:249-252.

20. Becker BB. Punctal occlusion and blepharoplasty in patients with dry eye syndrome. *Arch Otolaryngol Head Neck Surg.* 1991;117(7):789-791.

21. Foulks GN. 2007 report of the International Dry Eye WorkShop (DEWS). *Ocular Surf.* 2007;5(2):81-86.

22. Guillon M, Styles E, Guillon JP, Maissa C. Preocular tear film characteristics of nonwearers and soft contact lens wearers. *Optom Vis Sci.* 1997;74(5):273-279.

23. Henriquez AS, Korb DR. Meibomian glands and contact lens wear. *Br J Ophthalmol.* 1981;65(2):108-111.

24. Arita R, Itoh K, Inoue K, et al. Contact lens wear is associated with decrease of meibomian glands. *Ophthalmology.* 2009;116(3):379-384.

25. Hom MM, Bruce AS. Prelens tear stability: relationship to symptoms of dryness. *Optometry.* 2009;80(4):181-184.

26. Fuller D. Yes, dry eye patients can wear contacts. Review of Optometry. 2015;Aug 15.

27. Ramamoorthy P, Nichols JJ. Compliance factors associated with contact lens-related dry eye. *Eye Contact Lens.* 2014;40(1):17-22.

28. Chalmers R, Long B, Dillehay S, Begley C. Improving contact lens related dryness symptoms with silicone hydrogel lenses. *Optom Vis Sci.* 2008;85(8):778-784.

29. Tilia D, Lazon de la Jara P, Peng N, et al. Effect of lens and solution choice on the comfort of contact lens wearers. *Optom Vis Sci.* 2013;90(5):411-418.

30. Maruyama K, Yokoi N, Takamata A, Kinoshita S. Effect of environmental conditions on tear dynamics in soft contact lens wearers. *Invest Ophthalmol Vis Sci.* 2004;45:2563-2568.

31. Forister JF, Forister EF, Yeung KK, et al. Prevalence of contact lens-related complications: UCLA contact lens study. *Eye Contact Lens.* 2009;35:176-180.

32. US Food and Drug Administration. Colored and decorative contact lenses: a prescription is a must. FDA Consumer Health Information. February 2016.

33. Sauer A, Bourcier T. Microbial keratitis as a foreseeable complication of cosmetic contact lenses: a prospective study. *Acta Ophthalmol.* 2011;89:439-442.

34. Young G, Young AG, Lakkis C, et al. Review of complications associated with contact lenses from unregulated sources of supply. *Eye Contact Lens.* 2014;40:58-64.

35. Hotta F Eguchi H, Imai S, et al. Scanning electron microscopy findings with energy-dispersive x-ray investigations of cosmetically tinted contact lenses. *Eye Contact Lens.* 2015;41(5):291-296.

36. Chan KY, Cho P, Boost M, et al. Microbial adherence to cosmetic contact lenses. *Cont Lens Anterior Eye.* 2014;37:267-272.

CHAPTER 7

A 62-Year-Old Postmenopausal Woman Diagnosed With Early Stage Glaucoma

The Role of Hormones, Age, and Topical Antihypertensives

Michelle J. Kim, MD and Preeya K. Gupta, MD

KEY POINTS

♦ Dry eye disease (DED) is more prevalent in women, tends to worsen with age, and is influenced by topical and systemic medications.

♦ More than 60% of patients on topical antihypertensives develop signs or symptoms suggestive of DED.

♦ Preservatives, such as benzalkonium chloride, are commonly used in topical glaucoma medications, which have been shown to result in tear film instability and disruption of the corneal epithelial barrier.

♦ Consider preservative-free formulations of topical glaucoma medications.

♦ Consider nonpharmacological options (selective laser trabeculoplasty or minimally invasive glaucoma surgical devices) in the treatment of concomitant glaucoma and DED.

A 62-year-old woman on topical glaucoma medications has several factors that predispose her to dry eye disease (DED). Both evaporative and aqueous deficient DED are more prevalent in women, tend to worsen with age, and are influenced by topical and systemic medications.[1] To effectively treat this population, the clinician needs to be aware of the additional elements at play and take a multifactorial approach to treating the disease.

Mah FS, Rhee MK, eds.
Dry Eye Disease: A Practical Guide (pp 67-72).
© 2019 Taylor & Francis Group.

AGING

In patients over 50 years old, the prevalence of DED has been estimated to be between 5% and 35%,[1-3] representing a significant disease burden with substantial socioeconomic implications. There are numerous pathophysiologic mechanisms at play, including alterations in the lacrimal functional unit, hyposecretion from the lacrimal glands, meibomian gland atrophy, reduction in corneal nerve density, tear film instability, imbalances of the immune system, reduced hormonal stimulation, development of conjunctivochalasis, and eyelid malposition.[4-6]

With age, there is also an increased prevalence of autoimmune conditions and inflammatory processes that are often comorbid with DED,[6] such as Sjögren syndrome, thyroid disease, rosacea, and blepharitis. Normal aging processes also herald mild immune dysregulation that can exacerbate DED. On a molecular level, the ocular surfaces of older patients with DED were found to have higher levels of CD4+ T cells with fewer anti-inflammatory regulatory T cells than their younger counterparts.[5] Furthermore, there are higher concentrations of inflammatory cytokines with elevated osmolarity. Cytokines such as interleukins 6 and 8 and tumor necrosis factor alpha exacerbate inflammation by recruiting additional inflammatory cells, while interferon gamma promotes goblet cell loss and conjunctival keratinization.[7,8] The build-up of these proinflammatory mediators then promotes further hyperosmolarity and inflammation, thus feeding the vicious cycle.

The mechanics of the lacrimal functional unit and the ocular surface may also amplify the inflammatory cycle. Eyelid malpositions such as involutional ectropion and entropion, horizontal laxity, lagophthalmos, and eyelid retraction not only prevent the effective drainage of inflammatory cytokines but also result in exposure keratopathy and irregular redistribution of the tear film with blinks. The effects of these eyelid malpositions are further exacerbated by a decreased blink rate with age. Unsurprisingly, it is estimated that more than 50% of patients with eyelid abnormalities experience clinically significant DED.[9] Conjunctivochalasis, or redundant folds in the conjunctiva, similarly disrupts the smooth distribution of the tear film and prolongs inflammatory mediators.[10] The prevalence of conjunctivochalasis has been estimated to be 98% in patients over 60 years old, making it a significant contributor to DED.[11]

Systemic medical disease and consequently polypharmacy become increasingly common with age. Multiple systemic medications, especially those with anticholinergic or dehydrating effects, are implicated in contributing to DED, including antidepressants, antihistamines, decongestants, multivitamins, and high-dose aspirin.[2,3] Other conditions that were found to increase the risk of dry eye include osteoarthritis, osteoporosis, history of previous fractures, and previous cataract surgery.[2]

Going back to our patient, a thorough ocular examination and medical history should be obtained to determine whether any of these additional risk factors with aging are present. Review of systems should be performed to identify symptoms that may be suggestive of autoimmune or musculoskeletal disorders. The patient's medication list should be reviewed to assess potentially offending medications. Finally, in addition to the standard testing for DED, a dynamic examination of lacrimal functional unit should be done, carefully noting the presence of eyelid abnormalities or conjunctivochalasis.

TOPICAL ANTIHYPERTENSIVES

In addition to the other changes with aging noted previously, glaucoma also becomes more prevalent with age. The use of one or more topical antihypertensives can exacerbate DED, and it has been estimated that more than 60% of patients on topical antihypertensives develop signs or symptoms suggestive of DED.[12] Patients on 2 or 3 topical medications, as is frequently the case, have increasingly worse dry eye symptoms.[13] Topical antihypertensives have been shown to increase tear film osmolarity[14] and accelerate meibomian gland atrophy as demonstrated on meibography.[15] Preservatives, such as benzalkonium chloride,[16] are commonly used in topical glaucoma medications, which have been shown to result in tear film instability and disruption of the corneal epithelial barrier.[6] In more severe cases, preservatives may lead to conjunctival scarring and forniceal foreshortening,[17] further disrupting the ocular surface.

Since our patient was diagnosed with early stage glaucoma, she may have been started on topical antihypertensive agents. She should be counseled on the contribution of glaucoma medications to DED and the availability of preservative-free formulations should the current agents worsen her dry eye symptoms. Additional nonpharmacological options such as selective laser trabeculoplasty or minimally invasive glaucoma surgical devices should be considered, especially in glaucoma patients with DED.

HORMONES

Women have a higher prevalence of DED than men, indicating that hormones may play a role in the regulation of the lacrimal functional unit.[1] After menopause, the sex steroid profile drastically changes. Estrogen levels experience a sharp decline, whereas androgens exhibit a steady decline that begins in adulthood and continues after menopause.[18,19] Androgens have been demonstrated to exert anti-inflammatory effects on the lacrimal and meibomian glands, with androgen deficiency leading to worse signs and symptoms of DED.[20,21] In contrast, the role of estrogens remains unclear and controversial,[20] with multiple reports of both higher and lower levels of estrogens contributing to dry eye symptoms.[22-24] These confounding reports may be due to the presence of differential estrogen receptors across different cell types on the ocular surface with variable affinity and activity depending on estrogen concentrations.[25] Therefore, the hormonal regulation of the ocular surface in women appears to be a complex process that still needs further investigation to be fully elucidated. Our patient should be asked if her dry eye symptoms changed after menopause, and whether she has previously used or is currently using any hormone replacement therapy (HRT).

TREATMENT CONSIDERATIONS

In addition to standard therapies for DED and meibomian gland dysfunction, special considerations should be taken in this patient. Preservative-free topical glaucoma medications have a similar efficacy profile for reducing intraocular pressure but do not alter the corneal epithelial barrier and produce fewer dry eye symptoms.[26] Depending on the severity of her symptoms, she should be prescribed preservative-free formulations of topical antihypertensives and artificial tears as well.

An additional measure to be discussed with her glaucoma specialist is whether she is a candidate for other pressure-lowering therapies, such as laser trabeculoplasty. Selective laser trabeculoplasty is a viable first-line agent for the treatment of glaucoma and produces pressure-lowering effects similar to that of one topical agent.[27] In some cases, this may obviate the need for years of topical therapy.

Since ocular surface inflammation tends to play a larger role with aging and postmenopausal states, topical cyclosporine A 0.05% should be considered as a method of both decreasing inflammation and increasing tear production in the aging population.[28] Topical lifitegrast 5% is a new medication that inhibits T-cell activation and cytokine release, thereby halting the inflammatory cycle. It has been shown to be effective at treating the signs and symptoms of DED as early as 2 weeks after starting therapy.[29] If our patient is taking any systemic medications that may exacerbate DED, there should be a coordinated approach with the primary care physician to determine if any of these can be discontinued or substituted.

If any significant eyelid malpositions are present, an evaluation with an oculoplastics specialist may help restore proper function. If clinically significant conjunctivochalasis is present, conjunctival resection or cautery can be considered, although care should be taken in a glaucoma patient to not excessively disrupt the conjunctiva in case of needed future glaucoma surgery.

Given the contribution of hormonal imbalances to DED, HRT may be considered. However, reports of such an approach are controversial. Multiple formulations of HRT exist, and there is currently no head-to-head comparison of the different types. Transdermal estrogen may worsen dry eye symptoms,[30] whereas transdermal testosterone has been reported to have no effect in one study[30] while in another led to significant improvements in tear break-up time, Schirmer test, and the Ocular Surface Disease Index questionnaire.[31] A small retrospective study of patients already on HRT with esterified estrogen and methyltestosterone reported significant improvements in dry eye symptoms.[32] A randomized controlled trial of oral estrogen and medroxyprogesterone identified an improvement in the Schirmer test in the treatment group but only for patients under 50 years old.[33] Yet another HRT regimen consisting of oral estradiol for 14 days followed by oral estradiol and dydrogesterone (a synthetic progesterone) for the subsequent 14 days found an improvement in dry eye symptoms, severity of eyelid meibomian disease, and corneal staining in perimenopausal women.[34] Therefore, there is no consensus on the formulation, route, or duration of HRT that is needed to produce symptomatic improvement of DED. In light of the potential negative side effects of HRT, such as the gynecologic malignancies and thromboembolism, the decision to start such a treatment must be individualized and carefully considered in conjunction with the primary care physician or gynecologist.

SUMMARY

This 62-year-old postmenopausal woman diagnosed with early stage glaucoma has DED that is complex and multifactorial in nature. Therefore, a single-pronged approach is insufficient for therapy. The contributions of hormonal imbalances, normal alterations in the ocular surface immunity with aging, systemic comorbidities, topical and systemic medications, eyelid abnormalities, and glaucoma therapy should be taken into account. Especially paramount treatment considerations in this age group include using preservative-free formulations of all topical agents whenever possible, discontinuation or substitution of systemic medications that may be contributing, the correction of eyelid or conjunctival abnormalities that lead to irregular distribution of the tear film, the initiation of topical anti-inflammatory agents such as cyclosporine A 0.05% or lifitegrast 5%, and the careful consideration of HRT. Such a multipronged approach will combat the various pathophysiologic mechanisms that cause DED in this population.

REFERENCES

1. The epidemiology of dry eye disease: report of the Epidemiology Subcommittee of the International Dry Eye WorkShop (2007). *Ocul Surf.* 2007;5(2):93-107.
2. Moss SE, Klein R, Klein BE. Prevalence of and risk factors for dry eye syndrome. *Arch Ophthalmol.* 2000;118(9):1264-1268.
3. Moss SE, Klein R, Klein BE. Long-term incidence of dry eye in an older population. *Optom Vis Sci.* 2008;85(8):668-674.
4. Gipson IK. Age-related changes and diseases of the ocular surface and cornea. *Invest Ophthalmol Vis Sci.* 2013;54(14):ORSF48-53.
5. Farid M, Agrawal A, Fremgen D, et al. Age-related Defects in Ocular and Nasal Mucosal Immune System and the Immunopathology of Dry Eye Disease. *Ocul Immunol Inflamm.* 2016;24(3):327-347.
6. Sharma A, Hindman HB. Aging: a predisposition to dry eyes. *J Ophthalmol.* 2014;2014:781683.
7. Lam H, Bleiden L, de Paiva CS, et al. Tear cytokine profiles in dysfunctional tear syndrome. *Am J Ophthalmol.* 2009;147(2):198-205 e1.
8. Massingale ML, Li X, Vallabhajosyula M, et al. Analysis of inflammatory cytokines in the tears of dry eye patients. *Cornea.* 2009;28(9):1023-1027.
9. Damasceno RW, Osaki MH, Dantas PE, Belfort R, Jr. Involutional ectropion and entropion: clinicopathologic correlation between horizontal eyelid laxity and eyelid extracellular matrix. *Ophthal Plast Reconstr Surg.* 2011;27(5):321-326.
10. Di Pascuale MA, Espana EM, Kawakita T, Tseng SC. Clinical characteristics of conjunctivochalasis with or without aqueous tear deficiency. *Br J Ophthalmol.* 2004;88(3):388-392.
11. Mimura T, Yamagami S, Usui T, et al. Changes of conjunctivochalasis with age in a hospital-based study. *Am J Ophthalmol.* 2009;147(1):171-177e1.
12. Leung EW, Medeiros FA, Weinreb RN. Prevalence of ocular surface disease in glaucoma patients. *J Glaucoma.* 2008;17(5):350-355.
13. Fechtner RD, Godfrey DG, Budenz D, et al. Prevalence of ocular surface complaints in patients with glaucoma using topical intraocular pressure-lowering medications. *Cornea.* 2010;29(6):618-621.

14. Lee SY, Wong TT, Chua J, et al. Effect of chronic anti-glaucoma medications and trabeculectomy on tear osmolarity. *Eye (Lond).* 2013;27(10):1142-1150.

15. coma medications on meibomian glands. *Cornea.* 2012;31(11):1229-1234.

16. Tomic M, Kastelan S, Soldo KM, Salopek-Rabatic J. Influence of BAK-preserved prostaglandin analog treatment on the ocular surface health in patients with newly diagnosed primary open-angle glaucoma. *Biomed Res Int.* 2013;2013:603782.

17. Schwab IR, Linberg JV, Gioia VM, Benson WH, Chao GM. Foreshortening of the inferior conjunctival fornix associated with chronic glaucoma medications. *Ophthalmology.* 1992;99(2):197-202.

18. Burger HG, Hale GE, Robertson DM, Dennerstein L. A review of hormonal changes during the menopausal transition: focus on findings from the Melbourne Women's Midlife Health Project. *Hum Reprod Update.* 2007;13(6):559-565.

19. Al-Azzawi F, Palacios S. Hormonal changes during menopause. Maturitas. 2009;63(2):135-137.

20. Sullivan DA. Tearful relationships? Sex, hormones, the lacrimal gland, and aqueous-deficient dry eye. *Ocul Surf.* 2004;2(2):92-123.

21. Krenzer KL, Dana MR, Ullman MD, et al. Effect of androgen deficiency on the human meibomian gland and ocular surface. *J Clin Endocrinol Metab.* 2000;85(12):4874-4882.

22. Gagliano C, Caruso S, Napolitano G, et al. Low levels of 17-beta-oestradiol, oestrone and testosterone correlate with severe evaporative dysfunctional tear syndrome in postmenopausal women: a case-control study. *Br J Ophthalmol.* 2014;98(3):371-376.

23. Shen G, Ma X. High Levels of 17beta-Estradiol Are Associated with Increased Matrix Metalloproteinase-2 and Metalloproteinase-9 Activity in Tears of Postmenopausal Women with Dry Eye. *J Ophthalmol.* 2016;2016:2415867.

24. Golebiowski B, Badarudin N, Eden J, et al. Does endogenous serum oestrogen play a role in meibomian gland dysfunction in postmenopausal women with dry eye? *Br J Ophthalmol.* 2016.

25. Versura P, Giannaccare G, Campos EC. Sex-steroid imbalance in females and dry eye. *Curr Eye Res.* 2015;40(2):162-175.

26. de Jong C, Stolwijk T, Kuppens E, de Deizer R, van Best J. Topical timolol with and without benzalkonium chloride: epithelial permeability and autofluorescence of the cornea in glaucoma. Graefes Arch *Clin Exp Ophthalmol.* 1994;232:221-224.

27. Katz LJ, Steinmann WC, Kabir A, et al. Selective laser trabeculoplasty versus medical therapy as initial treatment of glaucoma: a prospective, randomized trial. *J Glaucoma.* 2012;21(7):460-468.

28. Ezuddin NS, Alawa KA, Galor A. Therapeutic strategies to treat dry eye in an aging population. *Drugs Aging.* 2015;32(7):505-513.

29. Holland EJ, Luchs J, Karpecki PM, et al. Lifitegrast for the treatment of dry eye disease: results of a phase III, randomized, double-masked, placebo-controlled trial (OPUS-3). *Ophthalmology.* 2017;124(1):53-60.

30. Golebiowski B, Badarudin N, Eden J, et al. The effects of transdermal testosterone and oestrogen therapy on dry eye in postmenopausal women: a randomised, placebo-controlled, pilot study. *Br J Ophthalmol.* 2016.

31. Nanavaty MA, Long M, Malhotra R. Transdermal androgen patches in evaporative dry eye syndrome with androgen deficiency: a pilot study. *Br J Ophthalmol.* 2014;98(4):567-569.

32. Scott G, Yiu SC, Wasilewski D, Song J, Smith RE. Combined esterified estrogen and methyltestosterone treatment for dry eye syndrome in postmenopausal women. *Am J Ophthalmol.* 2005;139(6):1109-1110.

33. Feng Y, Feng G, Peng S, Li H. The effects of hormone replacement therapy on dry eye syndromes evaluated by Schirmer test depend on patient age. *Cont Lens Anterior Eye.* 2016;39(2):124-127.

34. Jin X, Lin Z, Liu Y, Lin L, Zhu B. Hormone replacement therapy benefits meibomian gland dysfunction in perimenopausal women. *Medicine (Baltimore).* 2016;95(31):e4268.

Chapter 8

Floppy Eyelid Syndrome

Kelsey Roelofs, MD and Audrey A. Chan, MD, FRCSC

Key Points

- Floppy eyelid syndrome (FES) is more common in overweight men, 40 to 69 years old.
- Typical presenting symptoms include eyelid swelling, ocular surface discomfort, conjunctival injection, mucoid discharge, and tearing; often worse on the dominant sleep side, particularly in the morning.
- Typical signs include profound eyelid laxity, papillary conjunctivitis, and punctate epithelial keratopathy.
- There is a well-documented association of FES with obstructive sleep apnea (OSA), which is linked with other medical comorbidities, such as hypertension and increased cardiovascular risk. Eighty-five percent of patients with FES have OSA.
- Treatment includes lubrication, eyelid taping and/or use of an eye shield at night, continuous positive airway pressure therapy, and eyelid tightening procedures.

Mah FS, Rhee MK, eds.
Dry Eye Disease: A Practical Guide (pp 73-83).
© 2019 Taylor & Francis Group.

Figure 8-1. Middle-aged man with upper eyelid that everts easily with minimal horizontal traction.

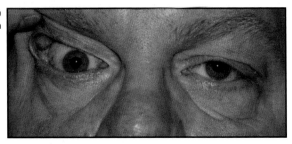

"My Eye Hurts and My Wife Says That I Snore"

A 52-year-old man presents with a chief complaint of a 2-month duration of irritation and soreness in the right eye. He experiences a gritty sensation, burning, and tearing in the eyes, particularly worse on the right side. He states that he rubs his eyes vigorously to relieve the sensation in the morning. He has been waking up with stringy discharge in the right eye recently. Lubricating eye drops and over-the-counter anti-allergy oral medication have been tried without significant relief.

His past medical history is significant for obesity, hypertension, and hyperlipidemia. On further questioning, he states that his wife does tell him that he snores, and he is often drowsy during the daytime.

Ocular examination reveals significant upper and lower eyelid laxity with easy eversion of the upper tarsal plate with horizontal tension (Figure 8-1). Blepharoptosis, particularly laterally, and eyelash ptosis are also noted. The palpebral conjunctiva shows papillary conjunctivitis, and there is course diffuse epithelial staining with fluorescein. The remainder of his anterior segment and dilated funduscopic examination is unremarkable.

This patient's history and examination are consistent with a diagnosis of floppy eyelid syndrome (FES). He was referred for a sleep study and was diagnosed with obstructive sleep apnea (OSA). Management of his ocular complaints initially included ointment lubrication and eye shield use at nighttime, which he felt did improve his symptoms but was inconvenient. He eventually had a eyelid shortening procedure on his right upper eyelid, which resolved his symptoms definitively.

This chapter explores the presentation, diagnosis, associations, and treatment of FES.

Introduction

FES was first described by Culbertson and Ostler in 1981.[1] They stated that:

> The most distinctive feature in each case was the rubbery, malleable upper tarsus. Any external upward force applied gently to the upper eyelid caused the tarsus to evert … none of the patients were aware of any previous ocular disease. In all cases, large papillae covered the upper palpebral conjunctiva.[1]

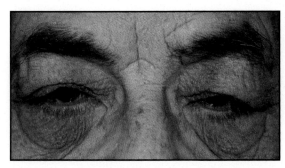

Figure 8-2. Characteristic associated findings of blepharochalasis, blepharoptosis, eyelash ptosis, and bilateral lower eyelid ectropion in a patient with FES.

Although all the patients studied in this sentinel paper on FES were overweight, middle-aged men,[1] we now know that women and non-obese patients can be affected, although much less commonly.[2] FES is an underdiagnosed and an often forgotten cause of the red, chronically irritated eye.[3] Herein, we will discuss a rational approach to the diagnosis and management of patients with FES.

A RATIONAL APPROACH TO THE DIAGNOSIS OF FLOPPY EYELID SYNDROME

History

FES is more common in men, 40 to 69 years old[2,4]; however, it can affect women and children, albeit much less commonly. Typical presenting symptoms of patients with FES include eyelid swelling, foreign body sensation/ocular surface discomfort, conjunctival injection, mucoid discharge, photosensitivity, and tearing.[4-7] These complaints may be unilateral or bilateral[6,8] and are often worse on the dominant sleep side, particularly in the morning owing to contact of the palpebral conjunctiva with the pillow during sleep.[9] Obesity is associated with FES,[1,2,4,6] and patients often have a positive history of habitual eye rubbing.[10]

It is essential to obtain a sleep history, asking about snoring and observed episodes of apnea. There is a well-documented association of FES with OSA, as we will discuss in depth later in this chapter.

Ocular Examination

A number of characteristic signs may be identified when examining a patient with FES, but perhaps the most defining of all is the profound laxity of the patient's upper eyelids, allowing for significant distraction from the globe along with a propensity for the eyelids to evert. Evaluation of the tear film and ocular surface in patients with FES will often reveal decreased Schirmer scores[1] as well as rapid tear break-up time.[12] Examination of the eyelids may be notable for eyelash ptosis,[2,13] loss of eyelash parallelism,[14] dermatochalasis,[2,15] and occasionally blepharoptosis (Figure 8-2).[10] Conjunctival

TABLE 8-1

DIAGNOSIS OF FLOPPY EYELID SYNDROME	
Epidemiology	**Ocular Findings**
40 to 69 years old	Profound eyelid laxity
Men more than women	Blepharoptosis
Overweight	Eyelash ptosis
Symptoms	Papillary conjunctivitis
Foreign body sensation	Decreased tear break-up time
Ocular irritation	Punctate epithelial keratopathy
Tearing	Corneal abrasions
Stringy discharge	Corneal neovascularization
Photosensitivity	Meibomian gland dysfunction
Spontaneous eyelid eversion	**Associated Diseases**
	Obstructive sleep apnea
	Keratoconus
	Non-arteritic ischemic optic neuropathy
	Glaucoma
	Recurrent corneal erosions
	Central serous chorioretinopathy

and corneal inspection shows a papillary reaction on the upper palpebral conjunctiva,[1,16] superficial punctate keratopathy,[17] and in more advanced cases, corneal neovascularization,[16] scarring,[2] and even thinning with possible perforation.[18] Moreover, other corneal conditions, such as keratoconus, are seen more commonly in patients with FES.[17,19] Blepharitis and meibomian gland dysfunction are often seen in patients with FES,[8] and some hypothesize that meibomianitis may be implicated in the pathogenesis of FES.[7,20]

Several methods for categorizing the degree of eyelid laxity have been described, including measurement of the amount of anterior distraction of the upper eyelid. Iyengar and Khan concluded that in patients with FES, their upper eyelid was able to be distracted a mean of 17 mm anteriorly from the globe.[21] They further commented that the magnitude of upper eyelid distraction correlated well with disease symptomatology.[21]

The diagnosis of FES is made clinically through identification of characteristic presentation and examination findings (Table 8-1). Though more defined criteria have been proposed to narrow the definition of FES, at this time, there is no widely accepted formal diagnostic criteria for FES. It should always be considered in patients presenting with the aforementioned complaints and with lax eyelids, while keeping in mind its differential diagnosis (Table 8-2).

TABLE 8-2

DIFFERENTIAL DIAGNOSIS OF FLOPPY EYELID SYNDROME

Dry Eye Syndrome

  Aqueous tear deficiency

  Meibomian gland dysfunction

Ocular Surface Inflammatory Disorders

  Atopic keratoconjunctivitis

  Superior limbic keratoconjunctivitis

  Allergic conjunctivitis

  Giant papillary conjunctivitis

Corneal Disorders

  Anterior basement membrane dystrophy

  Salzmann nodular degeneration

Eyelid and Eyelash Disorders

  Entropion

  Ectropion

  Trichiasis

  Chalazion

Miscellaneous

  Conjunctival foreign body under upper eyelid

  Conjunctivitis medicamentosa (particularly secondary to chronic use of topical eye drops containing vasoconstrictive agents)

HISTOPATHOLOGY

Several studies have performed histopathological examination of eyelid tissue from patients with FES. Compared to healthy individuals, there is a decreased amount of mature elastin fibers in the tarsus of patients with FES,[10,22] and one study found an increased abundance of oxytalan fibers.[22] In addition to chronic inflammation and decreased quantity of elastin fibers, increased expression of elastin-degrading enzymes, matrix metalloproteinase (MMP-7 and MMP-9), is found in FES.[16]

Some studies have concluded that the amount and quality of tarsal collagen is within normal limits in FES.[10] Others have noted an increased amount of type 1 and 3 collagen within the tarsal plate of patients with FES, stating that this change is consistent with an adaptive response to repetitive mechanical trauma to the tarsal plate.[22]

PATHOPHYSIOLOGY

Several theories have been proposed to explain the pathophysiological mechanisms by which FES ensues.

Mechanical Trauma

Repeated mechanical trauma from eversion and irritation of the eyelid during sleep is the prevailing theory behind the cause of FES. When the patient with lax eyelids sleeps face down, the eyelid is prone to becoming everted and rubbing on the pillow,[2] resulting in commencement of a chronic cycle of irritation. This theory is supported by the fact that many patients note worse symptoms on the side that they sleep on.[19] Histopathologically, this hypothesis is supported by the finding that elastolytic enzymes (MMP-7 and MMP-9) are induced by repeated mechanical stress and have been found to be upregulated in FES, subsequently leading to further elastic fiber degeneration and resultant progression of tarsal laxity and eyelash ptosis.[16]

Ischemia-Reperfusion Injury

Some have suggested that given the strong association between FES and OSA, repetitive episodes of systemic hypoxia secondary to apneic events, followed by reperfusion of the tarsal plate when the patient begins breathing normally again, may result in the release of free radicals. It is then postulated that this free radical release results in damage to the tarsal stroma and stimulation of a papillary conjunctivitis. However, given that the tarsal plate has a very low oxygen demand, this theory may be less likely.[2]

Genetic Predisposition

Some authors have suggested that an underlying genetic predisposition to collagen and/or elastin abnormality may play an important role in the pathogenesis of FES.[23] While there is a paucity of literature reporting a specific genetic predisposition in the pathophysiology of FES, there have been significant genome-level findings documenting genetic risk loci for OSA.[24]

SYSTEMIC ASSOCIATIONS

While overall, the incidence of FES among all patients diagnosed with OSA has been reported to be quite low (2.3%),[25] a significant proportion (85%) of patients with FES have OSA.[26] Furthermore, as the severity of OSA increases, the incidence of FES rises,[27] and those with more severe OSA are more likely to have more severe FES.[26,28] Similarly, in patients with worse OSA, Schirmer and tear break-up time scores are decreased more significantly than in those with milder OSA.[11]

Some have proposed that the etiological link between FES and OSA lies in decreased elastic fibers in both the tarsal plate as well as the uvular tissue. This association is an important one for the clinician to identify, as patients with FES should be referred to a sleep physician to investigate for OSA.[29]

OSA occurs in an estimated 2% of women and 4% of men and is associated with obesity.[30] Daytime sleepiness is the most common presenting symptom; however, snoring may precede other symptoms by up to 15 years.[31] Sleep apnea is an important condition to identify, diagnose, and treat, as it is associated with other medical comorbidities, including hypertension and subsequent increased cardiovascular risk,[32] and these patients are at an increased risk of automobile accidents.[33]

In children with lax eyelids, other congenital associations, such as Down syndrome,[34] Ehlers-Danlos syndrome,[35] and congenital cataracts facial dysmorphism neuropathy syndrome,[36] should be carefully considered before diagnosing an acquired entity, such as FES.

OCULAR ASSOCIATIONS

Nonarteritic ischemic optic neuropathy, glaucoma, keratoconus, central serous chorioretinopathy, and recurrent corneal erosions[9,37] have all been found to be associated with OSA. Given the significant overlap in patient demographics between FES and OSA, the astute clinician will be mindful to examine for and rule in/out any of these associated ocular conditions in the patient presenting with FES.

Optic Neuropathies

It is theorized that patients with OSA are at higher risk for nonarteritic ischemic optic neuropathy due to impaired optic nerve head autoregulatory blood flow as a result of recurrent episodes of hypoxia secondary to apneic events leading to ischemia of the optic nerve head.[9] Additionally, the prevalence of glaucoma in patients with OSA and FES may be up to 23%. It is similarly proposed that episodic impairment in perfusion and oxygenation to the optic nerve head, as a result of apneic events, results in a glaucomatous optic neuropathy.[38]

Keratoconus

Keratoconus has been found to occur more frequently in patients with OSA[39] and also directly with FES.[19] Moreover, studies of patients with keratoconus have concluded that these patients have an increased propensity to have lax eyelids along the FES spectrum.[17] It has been hypothesized that this association may be due to changes in corneal biomechanical properties, as patients with FES appear to have significantly lower corneal hysteresis values, which may increase the propensity for ectasia.[40] Finally, eye rubbing is both an associated clinical finding in FES[10] and a risk factor for the development of keratoconus,[41] thus providing another mechanistic link between the 2 diseases.

MEDICAL TREATMENT

A variety of conservative measures can be attempted to improve the ocular surface of patients with FES, including lubrication, eyelid taping, and/or use of an eye shield at night[8]; however, many patients find these solutions impractical and inconvenient.

In patients with concurrent OSA and FES, continuous positive airway pressure therapy (CPAP) may be helpful in treating both systemic findings and ocular surface problems. CPAP may improve Schirmer and tear break-up time scores[42] and also necessitates supine positioning, thereby avoiding mechanical trauma from the everted eyelid rubbing on the pillow.[43]

SURGICAL TREATMENT

When medical therapy fails to adequately control the patient's symptoms, eyelid surgery becomes the mainstay of treatment. While there are a number of surgical options, they are all aimed at correcting the excessive horizontal eyelid laxity that exists. Many patients have coexisting blepharoptosis, and it is recommended that the horizontal eyelid laxity be corrected prior to performing a ptosis-correcting surgery such as anterior levator advancement.

Lateral Tarsal Strip

A lateral tarsal strip can be performed for patients with FES to correct the upper eyelid laxity and can also be used to concurrently tighten the often coexisting lower eyelid laxity. Following surgical correction via lateral tarsal strip, the majority of patients have significant improvement in symptoms[44] and other secondary signs, including eyelash ptosis.[6]

Pentagonal Wedge Resection

The pentagonal wedge resection can be used to effectively address FES. In addition to patient reports of subjective improvement in symptomatology after surgical correction of eyelid laxity, impression cytology following wedge resection objectively shows improvement in cellular morphology and goblet cell count in the majority of patients.[45] Moreover, as patients with FES can also have concurrent blepharoptosis,[5,10] horizontal eyelid tightening by way of a full-thickness wedge resection generally results in a secondary improvement in ptosis.[46]

The usual amount resected to address FES is generous, typically 10 to 12 mm.[47] With regard to placement of the wedge resection, some advocate that a laterally placed resection may be blended into the eyelid crease to tighten the eyelid in an aesthetically minded way,[48] while others feel that in FES, the eyelid redundancy is located medially and therefore advocate for medial wedge placement.[4]

SUMMARY

FES is an important and often overlooked diagnosis that must be considered in patients presenting with red, irritated eyes. While stepwise management may begin with conservative measures aimed at improving the health of the ocular surface, definitive treatment often requires surgical correction of eyelid laxity by way of a pentagonal wedge resection or lateral tarsal strip. In patients with FES, a thorough eye examination should be completed to carefully rule out any associated ocular conditions, especially those that can be relatively asymptomatic at early stages, such as keratoconus and glaucoma. The astute clinician will appropriately refer patients with the diagnosis of FES to be investigated for OSA, keeping in mind that in addition to systemic benefits, treatment with CPAP has also been shown to improve ocular symptomatology.

REFERENCES

1. Culbertson W, Ostler H. The floppy eyelid syndrome. *Am J Ophthalmol.* 1981;92(4):568-575.
2. Ezra DG, Beaconsfield M, Collin R. Floppy eyelid syndrome: stretching the limits. *Surv Ophthalmol.* 2010;55(1):35-46.
3. Huerva V, Muniesa MJ, Ascaso FJ. Floppy eyelid syndrome in obstructive sleep apnea syndrome. *Sleep Med.* 2014;15(6):724-727.
4. Valenzuela AA, Sullivan TJ. Medial upper eyelid shortening to correct medial eyelid laxity in floppy eyelid syndrome: a new surgical approach. *Ophthalmic Plast Reconstr Surg.* 2005;21(4):259-263.
5. Mastrota K. Impact of floppy eyelid syndrome in ocular surface and dry eye disease. *Optom Vis Sci.* 2008;85(9):814-816. doi:10.1097/OPX.0b013e3181852777.
6. Viana GAP, Sant'Anna AE, Righetti F, Osaki M. Floppy eyelid syndrome. *Plast Reconstr Surg.* 2008;121(5):333e-334e.
7. Gonnering R, Sonneland P. Meibomian gland dysfunction in floppy eyelid syndrome. *Ophthalmic Plast Reconstr Surg.* 1987;3(2):99-103.
8. Moore M, Harrington J, McCulley J. Floppy eyelid syndrome. Management including surgery. *Ophthalmology.* 1986;93(2):184-188.
9. Abdal H, Pizzimenti JJ, Purvis CC. The eye in sleep apnea syndrome. *Sleep Med.* 2006;7(2):107-115.
10. Netland P, Sugrue S, Albert D, Shore J. Histopathologic features of the floppy eyelid syndrome. Involvement of tarsal elastin. *Ophthalmology.* 1994;101(1):174-181.
11. Acar M, Firat H, Acar U, Ardic S. Ocular surface assessment in patients with obstructive sleep apnea-hypopnea syndrome. *Sleep Breath.* 2013;17(2):583-588.
12. Liu DTS, Di Pascuale MA, Sawai J, Gao YY, Tseng SCG. Tear film dynamics in floppy eyelid syndrome. *Invest Ophthalmol Vis Sci.* 2005;46(4):1188-1194. doi:10.1167/iovs.04-0913.
13. Klapper S, Jordan D. Floppy eyelid syndrome. *Ophthalmology.* 1998;105(9):1582.
14. Langford JD, Linberg J V. A new physical finding in floppy eyelid syndrome. *Ophthalmology.* 1998;105(1):165-169. doi:10.1016/S0161-6420(98)91960-1.
15. Ezra DG, Beaconsfield M, Sira M, Bunce C, Wormald R, Collin R. The associations of floppy eyelid syndrome: a case control study. *Ophthalmology.* 2010;117(4):831-838.
16. Schlötzer-Schrehardt U, Stojkovic M, Hofmann-Rummelt C, Cursiefen C, Kruse FE, Holbach LM. The pathogenesis of floppy eyelid syndrome: involvement of matrix metalloproteinases in elastic fiber degradation. *Ophthalmology.* 2005;112(4):694-704.

17. Pihlblad MS, Schaefer DP. Eyelid laxity, obesity, and obstructive sleep apnea in keratoconus. *Cornea*. 2013;32(9):1232-1236.

18. Rossiter J, Ellingham R, Hakin K, Twomey J. Corneal melt and perforation secondary to floppy eyelid syndrome in the presence of rheumatoid arthritis. *Br J Ophthalmol*. 2002;86(4):483.

19. Culbertson W, Tseng S. Corneal disorders in floppy eyelid syndrome. *Cornea*. 1994;13(1):33-42.

20. van den Bosch WA, Lemij HG. The lax eyelid syndrome. *Br J Ophthalmol*. 1994;78(9):666-670.

21. Iyengar S, Khan J. Quantifying upper eyelid laxity in symptomatic floppy eyelid syndrome by measurement of anterior eyelid distraction. *Ophthalmic Plast Reconstr Surg*. 2007;23(3):255.

22. Ezra DG, Ellis JS, Gaughan C, et al. Changes in tarsal plate fibrillar collagens and elastic fibre phenotype in floppy eyelid syndrome. *Clin Exp Ophthalmol*. 2011;39(6):564-571.

23. Lee WJ, Kim JC, Shyn KH. Clinical evaluation of corneal diseases associated with floppy eyelid syndrome. *Korean J Ophthalmol*. 1996;10:116-121.

24. Cade BE, Chen H, Stilp AM, et al. Genetic associations with obstructive sleep apnea traits in Hispanic/Latino Americans. *Am J Respir Crit Care Med*. 2016;194(7):886-897.

25. Karger RA, White WA, Park WC, et al. Prevalence of floppy eyelid syndrome in obstructive sleep apnea-hypopnea syndrome. *Ophthalmology*. 2006;113(9):1669-1674. doi:10.1016/j.ophtha.2006.02.053.

26. Muniesa MJ, Huerva V, Sánchez-de-la-Torre M, Martínez M, Jurjo C, Barbé F. The relationship between floppy eyelid syndrome and obstructive sleep apnoea. *Br J Ophthalmol*. 2013;97(11):1387-1390.

27. Wang P, Yu DJ, Feng G, et al. Is floppy eyelid syndrome more prevalent in obstructive sleep apnea syndrome patients? *J Ophthalmol*. 2016;2016:1-9.

28. Chambe J, Laib S, Hubbard J, et al. Floppy eyelid syndrome is associated with obstructive sleep apnoea: a prospective study on 127 patients. *J Sleep Res*. 2012;21(3):308-315.

29. Diaper CJM. Wake up to floppy eyelid syndrome. *Br J Ophthalmol*. 2013;97(11):1363-1364.

30. Young T, Palta M, Dempsey J, Skatrud J, Weber S, Badr S. The occurrence of sleep-disordered breathing among middle-aged adults. *N Engl J Med*. 1993;328:1230-1235.

31. Kales A, Cadieux R, Bixler E. Severe obstructive sleep apnea I. Onset, clinical course and characteristics. *J Chronic Dis*. 1985;38(5):419-425.

32. Cai A, Wang L, Zhou Y, Chen J, Feng Y, Zhong Q. OS 33-08 Obstructive sleep apnea promotes cardiovascular risk in hypertensive populations: a cross-sectional study. *J Hypertens*. 2016;34. doi: 10.1097/01.hjh.0000501012.38472.98.

33. George C, Nickerson P, Hanly P, Millar T, Kryger M. Sleep apnoea patients have more automobile accidents. *Lancet*. 1987;1:447.

34. Tawfik HA. Floppy eyelid associated with Down syndrome. *Orbit*. 2013;32(5):347-347.

35. Segev F, Héon E, Cole WG, et al. Structural abnormalities of the cornea and lid resulting from collagen V mutations. *Invest Ophthalmol Vis Sci*. 2006;47(2):565-573.

36. Müllner-Eidenböck A, Moser E, Klebermass N, et al. Ocular features of the congenital cataracts facial dysmorphism neuropathy syndrome. *Ophthalmology*. 2004;111(7):1415-1423.

37. Huon LK, Liu SYC, Camacho M, Guilleminault C. The association between ophthalmologic diseases and obstructive sleep apnea: a systematic review and meta-analysis. *Sleep Breath*. 2016;20(4):1-10.

38. Muniesa M, Sánchez-de-la-Torre M, Huerva V, Lumbierres M, Barbé F. Floppy eyelid syndrome as an indicator of the presence of glaucoma in patients with obstructive sleep apnea. *J Glaucoma*. 2014;23(1):e81-e85.

39. West SD, Turnbull C. Eye disorders associated with obstructive sleep apnoea. *Curr Opin Pulm Med*. 2016;22:595-601.

40. Royo M, Ribot A, Sanchez-De-La-Torre M, Escanilla V, Campo C, Barbeilla F. Corneal biomechanical properties in floppy eyelid syndrome. *Cornea*. 2015;34(5):521-524.

41. Sugar J, Macsai MS. What causes keratoconus? *Cornea*. 2012;31(6):716-719.

42. Acar M, Firat H, Yuceege M, Ardic S. Long-term effects of PAP on ocular surface in obstructive sleep apnea syndrome. *Can J Ophthalmol*. 2014;49(2):217-221.
43. Kadyan A, Asghar J, Dowson L, Sandramouli S. Ocular findings in sleep apnoea patients using continuous positive airway pressure. *Eye (Lond)*. 2010;24(5):843-850. doi:10.1038/eye.2009.212.
44. Burkat CN, Lemke BN. Acquired lax eyelid syndrome. *Ophthalmic Plast Reconstr Surg*. 2005;21(1):52-58.
45. Medel R, Alonso T, Vela JI, Calatayud M, Bisbe L, García-Arumí J. Conjunctival cytology in floppy eyelid syndrome: objective assessment of the outcome of surgery. *Br J Ophthalmol*. 2009;93(4):513-517.
46. Mills DM, Meyer DR, Harrison AR. Floppy eyelid syndrome. Quantifying the effect of horizontal tightening on upper eyelid position. *Ophthalmology*. 2007;114(10):1932-1936.
47. Tanenbaum M. A rational approach to the patient with floppy/lax eyelids. *Br J Ophthalmol*. 1994;78:663-664.
48. Periman LM, Sires BS. Floppy eyelid syndrome: a modified surgical technique. *Ophthalmic Plast Reconstr Surg*. 2002;18(5):370-372.

CHAPTER 9

"My Eyes Feel Better When I'm in Florida on Vacation"

Sotiria Palioura, MD, PhD and Guillermo Amescua, MD

KEY POINTS

- Environmental and occupational factors play a role in dry eye disease.
- Using a humidifier, taking visual breaks, and being mindful of blink frequency can help reduce dry eye symptoms.
- Even minor environmental and behavioral modifications can have a significant positive impact on patient symptoms.

The diagnosis of dry eye disease (DED) is particularly challenging in patients with early or mild disease, who tend to show few signs on clinical exam, but complain of severe symptoms.[1-5] Though there are many tests available for the assessment of the objective signs of DED (eg, tear osmolarity, tear break-up time, ocular surface staining, Schirmer testing, meibomian gland grading), they tend to be less reliable in cases of mild DED and they correlate poorly with patient-reported symptoms. Thus, a significant number of such patients remain undiagnosed or are labeled as having excessive symptoms due to psychosocial issues without objective findings. Moreover, the few clinical signs in such borderline patients may reverse completely in the absence of environmental

Mah FS, Rhee MK, eds.
Dry Eye Disease: A Practical Guide (pp 85-93).
© 2019 Taylor & Francis Group.

Figure 9-1. This is a 54-year-old woman with excessive complaints of pain and discomfort. Her symptoms are worse at work or during long periods of reading time. Exam shows a quiet ocular surface, but mild to moderate meibomian gland dysfunction with rapid tear film evaporation.

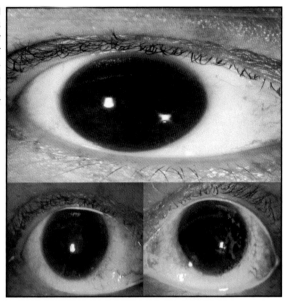

or occupational exposures such as low relative humidity or high-demanding visual display unit work that would normally exacerbate them. In such cases, it is not uncommon for the clinical exam to be "normal" and not representative of the actual disease.

Proper evaluation of dry eye patients, especially the ones with few signs and multiple symptoms, warrants investigation by the clinician of their personal, environmental, and occupational risk factors for temporary exacerbations of the disease. Personal risk factors that affect tear dynamics include age, gender, and the use of medications (eg, diuretics). Environmental risk factors that affect the stability of the tear film are temperature, relative humidity, wind/draft, outdoor air pollution, and allergens. Finally, occupational risk factors include time spent doing high concentration work on visual display units, indoor and/or outdoor air quality, and air particles (Figure 9-1).

PERSONAL RISK FACTORS

Aging

The quality of the lipid layer of the tear film gradually deteriorates with age.[6,7] In the meibum of children, lipid-lipid interactions are tighter and the concentration of total protein is higher than in adults.[6-8] The more unstable adult tear film is reflected by a higher blink frequency needed with advancing age[9,10] and a break-up time that is at least 3 times less than what is observed in children.[11,12] Incomplete blinks and eyelid malposition that occurs with age further destabilize an already-compromised tear film in adults.

Gender

Dry eye symptoms such as burning, irritation, discomfort, and stinging are known to be reported more by women than men.[13-16] Hormonal changes that come about with increasing age, use of cosmetic products, differences in the type of work, and psychological factors may account for a more unstable tear film in the case of women, which could explain the difference in dry eye incidence between the 2 groups. Changes in androgen and estrogen levels in aging women directly affect tear production by the lacrimal gland, thus causing deregulation of the homeostasis of the ocular surface. Lipophilic particles in cosmetics not only alter the lipid layer of the tear film but may migrate and change the aqueous-mucin layer as well.[17] Stress, depression, and a low sense of self-coherence have been associated with increasing reporting of dry eye symptoms in women,[18] whereas perceived work satisfaction decreases such reporting, even in the presence of objective findings of a destabilized tear film on clinical exam.[19]

Medications

Both systemic and topical medications can alter the homeostasis of the tear film, cause dry eye signs, and/or exacerbate dry eye symptoms.[20] Eye drops with the preservative benzalkonium chloride result in hyperosmolarity and instability of the tear film.[21] Though the exact mechanism of the effect on this preservative on the ocular surface remains unknown, benzalkonium chloride is able to penetrate deep into the cornea, conjunctiva, and even sclera in animal models.[22] Many systemic medications are known to alter lacrimal gland secretion, thus leading to the aqueous-deficient form of DED, including antidepressants, diuretics, antihistamines, and anti-androgens.[23-25]

ENVIRONMENTAL RISK FACTORS

Temperature

The effects of temperature on the stability of the tear film have been shown to be multifactorial. The TRPM8-dependent thermoreceptors present in the cornea play a role both in regulating basal tear production and blink frequency. Higher temperature reduces tear production[26] and lower temperature stimulates it. In an office setting, a 1°C decrease in the ambient temperature (within the 22°C to 26°C range) resulted in a 19% decrease of self-reported dry eye symptoms.[27] Similarly, stimulation of the cornea cold thermoreceptors triggers the blink reflex; in other words, cooler temperatures stimulate blinking.[28,29] A temperature higher than 25°C increases tear evaporation by at least 3-fold, which further destabilizes the precorneal tear film.[30,31] A higher temperature of the ocular surface renders the lipid layer of the tear film thicker by making the meibomian gland secretions more liquid-like. However, this is not enough to overcome the aforementioned effects of decreased basal tear production, decreased blink frequency, and increased evaporation rate. Thus, measurements of the tear break-up time are longer at lower rather than higher temperatures.[32,33]

Relative Humidity

Low relative humidity has been associated with a higher prevalence of dry eye symptoms.[34,35] Low humidity conditions increase the rate of tear evaporation causing instability of the tear film even in healthy volunteers.[36,37] In patients already diagnosed with DED, low relative humidity causes a higher blink frequency and more prominent fluorescein staining of the ocular surface.[38] Even in the presence of draft, which uniformly worsens dry eye symptoms, higher relative humidity (up to 74%) decreased self-reporting of ocular discomfort among healthy students.[39] Desiccation of the ocular surface increases the osmolarity of the tear film, which in turn stimulates an inflammatory cascade of events that bring about more epithelial damage,[40,41] either directly or indirectly through inadequate mucin production by the conjunctival goblet cells.[42]

Wind/Draft

Both horizontal and downward air velocity significantly increase tear evaporation rate.[31] The effects of a higher tear evaporation rate are not compensated for by the concomitant decrease in the temperature of the ocular surface or the increased blink frequency in patients with DED and an already unstable tear film.[43,44] In normal participants, the higher blink frequency and the lower corneal temperature stimulated by wind/draft overpower its desiccating effects and the tear meniscus measures higher than in lower draft conditions.[43]

Outdoor Air Particles

Nitrogen dioxide, ambient ozone, and particulate matter (eg, allergens) have all been shown to alter the precorneal tear film and, thus, to cause irritation and shortening of the break-up time.[45-49] A recent population-based epidemiological study with 16,824 participants showed that higher outdoor ozone levels and lower relative humidity correlate nicely with patient experience of dry eye symptoms and physician diagnosis of DED.[50] Reactive oxygen species and free radicals present in combustion particulate matter overwhelm the antioxidant defense mechanism of the ocular surface (eg, ascorbate, glutathione), thus leading to oxidative damage of the conjunctival goblet cells and the tear film.[51,52] Workers in the lower floors of office buildings are thought to experience more irritated and itchy eyes due to exposure to traffic combustion products.[53]

OCCUPATIONAL RISK FACTORS

Visual Display Unit Work

Visually and cognitively demanding tasks substantially reduce blink frequency and are associated with more incomplete blinks.[54-57] The more demanding the work visually and cognitively, the more dry eye symptoms ensue.[58,59] After such tasks, blink

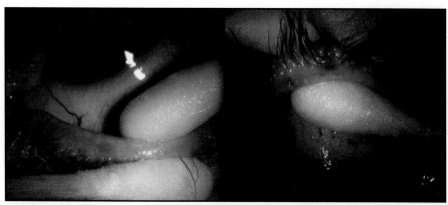

Figure 9-2. This is a 62-year-old woman with chronic ocular symptoms of dryness and irritation. Symptoms are worst in a low-humidity environment (flying, air condition). Ocular surface exam demonstrated normal corneal epithelium but significant stasis of her lower eyelid meibomian gland function.

frequency increases in an attempt to restore the tear film.[55] Screen positioning to eye level or below eye level may be preferable to minimize exposure-related dry eye.[55]

Indoor Air Particles

The measured concentrations of volatile organic compounds that are emitted by building materials and consumer products at baseline are too low to cause dry eye–related symptoms.[60] However, exposure to higher concentrations (eg, in areas close to construction sites) may intensify dry eye symptoms in patients with an already-compromised tear film. High-performance vacuuming that reduced the dust concentration to almost one-third of its baseline level led to significantly reduced irritation symptoms among office employees in at least 2 studies.[61]

MANAGEMENT PRINCIPLES

Modification of the aforementioned risk factors is crucial for the patient to experience improvement of his or her symptoms and the clinician to find less manifestations of the disease on clinical exam. The only modifiable personal risk factors are medications and psychosocial stress. Limited use of systemic medications that alter the tear film, use of eye drops without preservatives, and better stress coping mechanisms can have a role in restoring the stability of the tear film. Diet supplementation with omega-3 fatty acids is also essential for the protective function of the lipid layer of the tear film against desiccating conditions. Patients with meibomian gland dysfunction will also benefit from mechanical treatment of the gland to help prevent gland stasis that can lead to fibrosis of the gland (Figure 9-2). Environmental risk factors can be altered within a closed setting (eg, house or office), unless the patient moves to a different geographic area that is cooler, more humid, less windy, and with cleaner air. Within a closed setting, maintaining a lower room temperature, restoring a higher humidity level (eg, through use of a humidifier), having less air conditioning, and being away from traffic combustion products (eg, higher floors in an office building) can significantly improve dry eye symptoms. Finally, occupational risks can be minimized by taking frequent short breaks while performing highly demanding cognitive work on visual display units and being in an office setting where high performance vacuuming is regularly done.

SUMMARY

The evaluation and treatment of patients with DED can be challenging for the clinician because it is very common in daily clinical practice that patients express more symptoms and the clinical exam shows a healthy ocular surface or mild findings of DED. A complete ophthalmic evaluation of the cornea and ocular surface is mandatory in order to establish the severity and cause of these symptoms. A good clinical history can help the clinician find the etiology of the patient's signs and symptoms. Special emphasis on the personal, environmental, and occupational risk factors is necessary when the clinical exam is noncontributory. The classic clinical example is the patient who comes to the clinic for evaluation of eye discomfort and irritation and the clinical exam shows a quiet ocular surface. In these types of patients, it is particularly important to inquire about their job (eg, office work/visual display units). Frequently, these patients will mention that symptoms are improved during the weekend or while on vacation, especially when visiting places with relative high humidity. Identifying this environmental or occupational risk factor can help tailor the treatment plan. Even minor behavioral or lifestyle modifications can have a significant positive impact on patient symptomatology.

REFERENCES

1. Cuevas M, Gonzalez-Garcia MJ, Castellanos E, et al. Correlations among symptoms, signs, and clinical tests in evaporative-type dry eye disease caused by meibomian gland dysfunction (MGD). *Curr Eye Res.* 2012;37(10):855-863.
2. Nichols KK, Nichols JJ, Mitchell GL. The lack of association between signs and symptoms in patients with dry eye disease. *Cornea.* 2004;23(8):762-770.
3. Bron AJ, Tomlinson A, Foulks GN, et al. Rethinking dry eye disease: a perspective on clinical implications. *Ocul Surf.* 2014;12(2 Suppl):S1-S31.
4. Schmidl D, Witkowska KJ, Kaya S, et al. The association between subjective and objective parameters for the assessment of dry-eye syndrome. *Invest Ophthalmol Vis Sci.* 2015;56(3):1467-1472.
5. Sullivan BD, Crews LA, Messmer EM, et al. Correlations between commonly used objective signs and symptoms for the diagnosis of dry eye disease: clinical implications. *Acta Ophthalmol.* 2014;92(2):161-166.
6. Borchman D, Foulks GN, Yappert MC, Milliner SE. Changes in human meibum lipid composition with age using nuclear magnetic resonance spectroscopy. *Invest Ophthalmol Vis Sci.* 2012;53(1):475-482.
7. Mudgil P, Borchman D, Yappert MC, et al. Lipid order, saturation and surface property relationships: a study of human meibum saturation. *Exp Eye Res.* 2013;116:79-85.

8. Benlloch-Navarro S, Franco I, Sanchez-Vallejo V, Silvestre D, Romero FJ, Miranda M. Lipid peroxidation is increased in tears from the elderly. *Exp Eye Res*. 2013;115:199-205.

9. Sun WS, Baker RS, Chuke JC, et al. Age-related changes in human blinks. Passive and active changes in eyelid kinematics. *Invest Ophthalmol Vis Sci*. 1997;38(1):92-99.

10. Cruz AA, Garcia DM, Pinto CT, Cechetti SP. Spontaneous eyeblink activity. *Ocul Surf*. 2011;9(1):29-41.

11. Cho P, Brown B. Review of the tear break-up time and a closer look at the tear break-up time of Hong Kong Chinese. *Optom Vis Sci*. 1993;70(1):30-38.

12. Ozdemir M, Temizdemir H. Age- and gender-related tear function changes in normal population. *Eye (Lond)*. 2010;24(1):79-83.

13. McCarty CA, Bansal AK, Livingston PM, Stanislavsky YL, Taylor HR. The epidemiology of dry eye in Melbourne, Australia. *Ophthalmology*. 1998;105(6):1114-1119.

14. The epidemiology of dry eye disease: report of the Epidemiology Subcommittee of the International Dry Eye WorkShop (2007). *Ocul Surf*. 2007;5(2):93-107.

15. Uchino M, Schaumberg DA, Dogru M, et al. Prevalence of dry eye disease among Japanese visual display terminal users. *Ophthalmology*. 2008;115(11):1982-1988.

16. Schaumberg DA, Uchino M, Christen WG, Semba RD, Buring JE, Li JZ. Patient reported differences in dry eye disease between men and women: impact, management, and patient satisfaction. *PloS One*. 2013;8(9):e76121.

17. Malik A, Claoue C. Transport and interaction of cosmetic product material within the ocular surface: beauty and the beastly symptoms of toxic tears. *Cont Lens Anterior Eye*. 2012;35(6):247-259.

18. Runeson R, Norback D, Stattin H. Symptoms and sense of coherence: a follow-up study of personnel from workplace buildings with indoor air problems. *Int Arch Occup Environ Health*. 2003;76(1):29-38.

19. Kawashima M, Uchino M, Yokoi N, et al. Associations between subjective happiness and dry eye disease: a new perspective from the Osaka study. *PloS One*. 2015;10(4):e0123299.

20. Marshall LL, Roach JM. Treatment of dry eye disease. *The Consult Pharm*. 2016;31(2):96-106.

21. Wilson WS, Duncan AJ, Jay JL. Effect of benzalkonium chloride on the stability of the precorneal tear film in rabbit and man. *Br J Ophthalmol*. 1975;59(11):667-669.

22. Desbenoit N, Schmitz-Afonso I, Baudouin C, et al. Localisation and quantification of benzalkonium chloride in eye tissue by TOF-SIMS imaging and liquid chromatography mass spectrometry. *Anal Bioanal Chem*. 2013;405(12):4039-4049.

23. Tan LL, Morgan P, Cai ZQ, Straughan RA. Prevalence of and risk factors for symptomatic dry eye disease in Singapore. *Clin Exp Optom*. 2015;98(1):45-53.

24. Fraunfelder FT, Sciubba JJ, Mathers WD. The role of medications in causing dry eye. *J Ophthalmol*. 2012;2012:285851.

25. Sharma A, Hindman HB. Aging: a predisposition to dry eyes. *J Ophthalmol*. 2014;2014:781683.

26. Parra A, Madrid R, Echevarria D, et al. Ocular surface wetness is regulated by TRPM8-dependent cold thermoreceptors of the cornea. *Nat Med*. 2010;16(12):1396-1399.

27. Mendell MJ, Fisk WJ, Petersen MR, et al. Indoor particles and symptoms among office workers: results from a double-blind cross-over study. *Epidemiology*. 2002;13(3):296-304.

28. Collins M, Seeto R, Campbell L, Ross M. Blinking and corneal sensitivity. *Acta Ophthalmol (Copenh)*. 1989;67(5):525-531.

29. Mori A, Oguchi Y, Okusawa Y, Ono M, Fujishima H, Tsubota K. Use of high-speed, high-resolution thermography to evaluate the tear film layer. *Am J Ophthalmol*. 1997;124(6):729-735.

30. Abusharha AA, Pearce EI, Fagehi R. Effect of ambient temperature on the human tear film. *Eye Contact Lens*. 2016;42(5):308-312.

31. Borchman D, Foulks GN, Yappert MC, Mathews J, Leake K, Bell J. Factors affecting evaporation rates of tear film components measured in vitro. *Eye Contact Lens*. 2009;35(1):32-37.

32. Giraldez MJ, Naroo SA, Resua CG. A preliminary investigation into the relationship between ocular surface temperature and lipid layer thickness. *Cont Lens Anterior Eye*. 2009;32(4):177-180; quiz 193, 195.

33. Purslow C, Wolffsohn J. The relation between physical properties of the anterior eye and ocular surface temperature. *Optom Vis Sci*. 2007;84(3):197-201.

34. Azuma K, Ikeda K, Kagi N, Yanagi U, Osawa H. Prevalence and risk factors associated with nonspecific building-related symptoms in office employees in Japan: relationships between work environment, indoor air quality, and occupational stress. *Indoor Air*. 2015;25(5):499-511.

35. Wolkoff P. "Healthy" eye in office-like environments. *Environ Int.* 2008;34(8):1204-1214.

36. Madden LC, Tomlinson A, Simmons PA. Effect of humidity variations in a controlled environment chamber on tear evaporation after dry eye therapy. *Eye Contact Lens.* 2013;39(2):169-174.

37. Abusharha AA, Pearce EI. The effect of low humidity on the human tear film. *Cornea.* 2013;32(4):429-434.

38. Alex A, Edwards A, Hays JD, et al. Factors predicting the ocular surface response to desiccating environmental stress. *Invest Ophthalmol Vis Sci.* 2013;54(5):3325-3332.

39. Shan X, Zhou J, Chang VWC, Yang E-H. Comparing mixing and displacement ventilation in tutorial rooms: students' thermal comfort, sick building syndromes, and short-term performance. *Build Environ.* 2016;102:128-137.

40. Xiao B, Wang Y, Reinach PS, et al. Dynamic ocular surface and lacrimal gland changes induced in experimental murine dry eye. *PloS One.* 2015;10(1):e0115333.

41. Pelegrino FS, Pflugfelder SC, De Paiva CS. Low humidity environmental challenge causes barrier disruption and cornification of the mouse corneal epithelium via a c-jun N-terminal kinase 2 (JNK2) pathway. *Exp Eye Res.* 2012;94(1):150-156.

42. Corrales RM, de Paiva CS, Li DQ, et al. Entrapment of conjunctival goblet cells by desiccation-induced cornification. *Invest Ophthalmol Vis Sci.* 2011;52(6):3492-3499.

43. Koh S, Tung C, Kottaiyan R, Zavislan J, Yoon G, Aquavella J. Effect of airflow exposure on the tear meniscus. *J Ophthalmol.* 2012;2012:983182.

44. Nakamori K, Odawara M, Nakajima T, Mizutani T, Tsubota K. Blinking is controlled primarily by ocular surface conditions. *Am J Ophthalmol.* 1997;124(1):24-30.

45. Saxena R, Srivastava S, Trivedi D, Anand E, Joshi S, Gupta SK. Impact of environmental pollution on the eye. *Acta Ophthalmol Scand.* 2003;81(5):491-494.

46. Versura P, Profazio V, Cellini M, Torreggiani A, Caramazza R. Eye discomfort and air pollution. *Ophthalmologica.* 1999;213(2):103-109.

47. Bourcier T, Viboud C, Cohen JC, et al. Effects of air pollution and climatic conditions on the frequency of ophthalmological emergency examinations. *Br J Ophthalmol.* 2003;87(7):809-811.

48. Torricelli AA, Novaes P, Matsuda M, et al. Correlation between signs and symptoms of ocular surface dysfunction and tear osmolarity with ambient levels of air pollution in a large metropolitan area. *Cornea.* 2013;32(4):e11-e15.

49. Chang CJ, Yang HH, Chang CA, Tsai HY. Relationship between air pollution and outpatient visits for nonspecific conjunctivitis. *Invest Ophthalmol Vis Sci.* 2012;53(1):429-433.

50. Hwang SH, Choi YH, Paik HJ, Wee WR, Kim MK, Kim DH. Potential importance of ozone in the association between outdoor air pollution and dry eye disease in South Korea. *JAMA Ophthalmol.* 201 6 Mar 10. doi: 10.1001/jamaophthalmol.2016.0139. [Epub ahead of print]

51. Kuizenga A, van Haeringen NJ, Kijlstra A. Inhibition of hydroxyl radical formation by human tears. *Invest Ophthalmol Vis Sci.* 1987;28(2):305-313.

52. Rose RC, Richer SP, Bode AM. Ocular oxidants and antioxidant protection. *Proc Soc Exp Biol Med.* 1998;217(4):397-407.

53. Mendell MJ, Lei-Gomez Q, Mirer AG, Seppanen O, Brunner G. Risk factors in heating, ventilating, and air-conditioning systems for occupant symptoms in US office buildings: the US EPA BASE study. *Indoor Air.* 2008;18(4):301-316.

54. Chu CA, Rosenfield M, Portello JK. Blink patterns: reading from a computer screen versus hard copy. *Optom Vis Sci.* 2014;91(3):297-302.

55. Nielsen PK, Sogaard K, Skotte J, Wolkoff P. Ocular surface area and human eye blink frequency during VDU work: the effect of monitor position and task. *Eur J Appl Physiol.* 2008;103(1):1-7.

56. Portello JK, Rosenfield M, Chu CA. Blink rate, incomplete blinks and computer vision syndrome. *Optom Vis Sci.* 2013;90(5):482-487.

57. Argiles M, Cardona G, Perez-Cabre E, Rodriguez M. Blink rate and incomplete blinks in six different controlled hard-copy and electronic reading conditions. *Invest Ophthalmol Vis Sci.* 2015;56(11):6679-6685.

58. Gowrisankaran S, Nahar NK, Hayes JR, Sheedy JE. Asthenopia and blink rate under visual and cognitive loads. *Optom Vis Sci.* 2012;89(1):97-104.

59. Toomingas A, Hagberg M, Heiden M, Richter H, Westergren KE, Tornqvist EW. Risk factors, incidence and persistence of symptoms from the eyes among professional computer users. *Work.* 2014;47(3):291-301.

60. Wolkoff P. Indoor air pollutants in office environments: assessment of comfort, health, and performance. *Int J Hyg Environ Health.* 2013;216(4):371-394.

61. Skulberg KR, Skyberg K, Kruse K, et al. The effect of cleaning on dust and the health of office workers: an intervention study. *Epidemiology.* 2004;15(1):71-78.

CHAPTER 10

"I Had Gastric Bypass Surgery"

Alex Barsam, MD; Felipe A. Valenzuela, MD; and
Victor L. Perez, MD

KEY POINTS

- Vitamin A deficiency (VAD) is harmful to the ocular surface if left untreated and carries a high mortality rate in underdeveloped nations.
- It is critical to have a high suspicion level for VAD even in developed nations, as signs/symptoms and slit-lamp examination findings can mimic other ocular surface diseases, such as dry eye disease or exposure keratopathy.
- Adequate levels of essential fatty acids and Vitamin D are also necessary for optimizing the health of the ocular surface.

"I HAD GASTRIC BYPASS SURGERY"

A 44-year-old woman with a past history of obesity and dry eye disease presents for her yearly eye exam and states she still has a burning, gritty sensation in both of her eyes that has not improved with artificial tears. Aside from her visual complaints, she is elated about how much weight she has lost since her Roux-en-Y gastric bypass performed

Mah FS, Rhee MK, eds.
Dry Eye Disease: A Practical Guide (pp 95-107).
© 2019 Taylor & Francis Group.

3 years ago. On slit-lamp examination, her conjunctiva is dry and you notice a raised, foamy lesion near the temporal limbus bilaterally and +1 diffuse punctate epithelial erosions in both eyes. These erosions have worsened since her previous exam. At the end of the exam, she notes that she no longer feels comfortable driving at night and performing her daily activities due to the intermittent quality of her vision.

INTRODUCTION

Nutritional deficiencies following gastric bypass surgeries are common and are often a result of malabsorption of Vitamin B, folate, iron, zinc, calcium, and fat-soluble vitamins, such as Vitamins A, D, E, and K. Clinicians of all backgrounds should be aware of the potentially devastating visual consequences of malnutrition and malabsorption, as gastric bypass surgery is one of the most popular weight loss procedures with an estimated 200,000 bariatric surgeries performed each year in the United States alone.[1] Fat-soluble vitamin deficiency can take several months to years to develop postoperatively and can have significant effects on tear film constituents and ultimately the health of the ocular surface. This chapter focuses on these nutritional deficiencies that clinically impact the functional lacrimal unit, with specific focus on hypovitaminosis A.

VITAMIN A DEFICIENCY

It is well known that Vitamin A plays an important role in our vision and it is essential for the maintenance of healthy epithelium and tear film stability of the ocular surface. With this, it must be noted that Vitamin A deficiency (VAD) is the leading cause of preventable blindness in children worldwide, with an estimated 250,000 to 500,000 children affected.[2] Half of these children die within a year of losing their sight.[2] This is not just a problem for developing nations. In the developed world its incidence is on the rise, as bariatric surgery and the presence of underlying nonalcoholic steatohepatitis (NASH) are becoming more common.[3] Hypovitaminos A in the setting of dry eye pathology is known as *xerophthalmia*, and it has a multifactorial impact on the ocular surface.

Etiology

The etiology of VAD can include malnutrition, bariatric surgery, cystic fibrosis, anorexia nervosa, bulimia, alcoholism, dysphagia, colitis, intestinal malabsorption (eg, Crohn's disease), chronic pancreatitis, hookworm disease, and chronic cirrhosis.

Symptoms

Symptoms of VAD can include night blindness, bilateral discomfort, gritty sensation, blurred vision, decreased or intermittent visual acuity, and foreign body sensation.

TABLE 10-1

CLASSIFICATION SCHEME FOR ASSESSMENT OF XEROPHTHALMIA
Night blindness (XN)
Conjunctival xerosis (X1A)
Bitot's spots (X1B)
Corneal xerosis (X2)
Corneal ulceration/keratomalacia < one-third of corneal surface (X3A)
Corneal ulceration/keratomalacia > one-third of corneal surface (X3B)
Corneal scar (XS)
Xerophthalmia fundus (XF)
Adapted from Control of Vitamin A deficiency and xerophthalmia. WHO Technical Report Series, No. 672. Geneva, Switzerland: World Health Organization; 1982.

Signs

- Tear film: Low tear meniscus, decreased tear break-up time, abnormal Schirmer test.
- Conjunctiva: Dryness, wrinkling, foamy appearance, conjunctival xerosis or Bitot's spots.
- Cornea: Bilateral punctate epithelial erosions, plaque formation, stromal edema, sterile or infected ulcerations, perforation, necrosis.
- Fundus: Retinopathy, yellowish dots in the periphery.

XEROPHTHALMIA: BACKGROUND AND CLINICAL MANIFESTATIONS

This greek term (xerosis = dry, ophthalmia = inflamed eye) encompasses the constellation of ocular manifestations of hypovitaminosis A, from keratomalacia to night blindness (Table 10-1). VAD can have a wide spectrum of injury to the ocular surface, most of which are completely reversible with Vitamin A treatment. Prolonged, severe deficiency can present with limbal necrosis and/or corneal melt, which is ultimately irreversible. While malnutrition is the leading cause of VAD worldwide, in developed nations it is often a result of intense dieting, malabsorption, or chronic alcoholism.[4]

CONJUNCTIVAL XEROSIS (X1A)

Vitamin A–derived retinoids help regulate mucin production at the ocular surface, and as retinol stores are depleted, the transformation of keratinized epithelium to

Figure 10-1. Marked keratinization of the tarsal conjunctiva. (Reprinted with permission from Dr. Andrew J. Huang.)

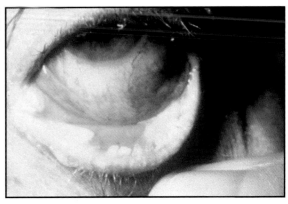

mucous-secreting columnar epithelium slows.[5] Metaplasia of the conjunctival epithelium to a stratified squamous type occurs, leading to a keratinized surface, and there is significant loss of mucin-secreting goblet cells.[6] The resulting keratinization of the ocular surface is what leads to the sandy, wrinkling, progressive drying of the conjunctiva, which can affect the tarsal conjunctiva as well (Figure 10-1). This process typically starts at the temporal limbus and sequentially involves the nasal, inferior, and superior limbus as the deficiency worsens.

Clinical Considerations

- Often a heaped up, whitish-foamy material that can be scraped off.
- Extent of xerosis correlates with degree of VAD.[7]
- Most xerosis will resolve 2 to 5 days after initiating Vitamin A replacement in young children.
- Must differentiate from other causes of xerosis/cicatrization.

BITOT'S SPOTS (X1B)

The conjunctival xerosis acts as a nidus for the build-up of meibomian secretions and keratin debris that can admix with a gas-producing bacterium, *Corynebacterium xerosis*, leading to the classic Bitot's spots (Figure 10-2A).[8] These lesions are often indicative of a past or present deficiency; however, Bitot's spots are sometimes observed in individuals with no supporting evidence of VAD, nor do the lesions always disappear with supplemental vitamin therapy.[8,9]

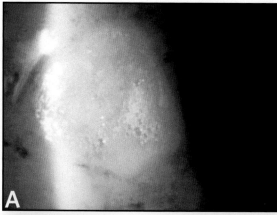

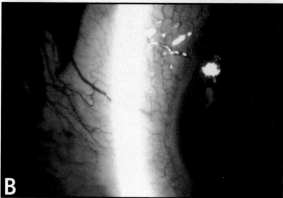

Figure 10-2. (A) Foamy, cheese-like Bitot's spot on conjunctiva. (Reprinted from *Cornea*, Mannis T, Mannis MJ, Paranjpe DR, Kirkness CM, 676-687, Copyright 2017, with permission from Elsevier.) (B) Bitot's spot on cornea. (Reprinted with permission from Dr. Andrew J. Huang.)

Clinical Considerations

- Foamy-appearing lesion that is triangularly shaped, bilateral, and will resolve with adequate replacement therapy in most cases.
- Can be seen on both conjunctiva and corneal surface (Figure 10-2B).
- Bitot's spots are not moisturized by tear film.
- Nasal lesions are a better indicator of active deficiency, although less prevalent.[6]
- Bitot's spots can persist for several weeks to months after systemic treatment.[10]

CORNEAL XEROSIS (X2)

Keratinization also plagues the surface of the cornea, leading to punctate keratopathy that can be easily identified with fluorescein stain. Corneal xerosis can be the earliest sign of VAD and can also represent prolonged, severe deficiency. Fortunately, it can respond rapidly to treatment.[11] Mild xerosis is characterized by corneal dryness and extensive areas of punctate keratopathy. Advanced xerosis presents as a haziness and

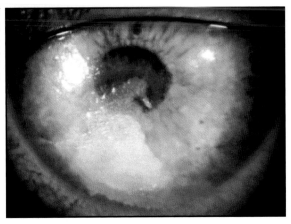

Figure 10-3. Keratinization of inferior cornea demonstrating "peau d'orange" appearance. (Reprinted from *Cornea*, Mannis T, Mannis MJ, Paranjpe DR, Kirkness CM, 676-687, Copyright 2017, with permission from Elsevier.)

roughness of the cornea from the build-up of keratin that is most prominent at the inferior borders of the cornea, which are more exposed. The keratinization can accumulate and eventually slough off, leaving behind a normal-appearing ocular surface. In more severe cases, the xerotic plaques can leave behind a corneal ulceration, as it strips away both basal epithelium and the underlying stroma.[12]

Clinical Considerations

- In mild xerosis, slit-lamp examination reveals superficial punctate keratopathy that stains with fluorescein and is most prominent inferonasally[11] and bilaterally.
- Negative-staining microcysts may also be present.
- In advanced xerosis, there will be more confluent keratinization, giving the corneal surface a lackluster, dry appearance with lack of corneal light reflex in the affected area.
- Classic "peau d'orange" appearance (Figure 10-3).
- Use a slit-lamp examination to identify focal areas of edema.
- Corneal findings can precede clinically detectable conjunctival xerosis, especially in abrupt deficiency (eg, measles).[7]

CORNEAL ULCERATION/KERATOMALACIA (X3A/X3B)

Ulceration resulting from VAD is usually a single, small, punched-out lesion with well-defined edges that often affects the peripheral cornea. Again, the spectrum of injury can vary from a single, partial-thickness ulceration, 1 to 2 mm in diameter, to a full-thickness perforation presenting as descemetocele. When Bowman's layer is compromised and proteolytic enzymes are released into the corneal stroma, liquefactive

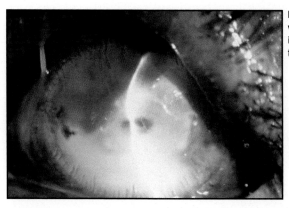

Figure 10-4. Severe keratomalacia with perforation and underlying infection. (Reprinted with permission from Dr. Andrew J. Huang.)

necrosis will occur, and ultimately lead to the sequelae of keratomalacia. This can be seen as limbus-to-limbus destruction and necrosis. Patients at this stage are at high risk of a superimposed infection (Figure 10-4), yet treatment necessitates Vitamin A repletion, as antibiotics do not prevent the ulceration or scar formation that can occur in VAD.[13]

Clinical Considerations

- Often a single, isolated ulcer in affected eye, often located inferonasally. Superficial ulcerations usually resolve without scar formation.
- Deeper ulcerations can perforate, but leaks are infrequent as the iris plugs the anterior chamber.[2]
- Ulceration can be accompanied by inflammation; hypopyon is seen in approximately 20% of cases.[6]
- Keratomalacia can present as a yellow or gray ulceration and can encompass the entire corneal surface.
- With treatment, gray lesions can heal with borders shrinking to an area smaller than the initial area affected.[10]
- Bitot's spots often show absence of fluorescein staining (negative staining), but can progress to positive staining just days after treatment initiation as the spot falls off.[14]

Critical

Vision is typically salvaged by treatment in cases where less than one-third of the cornea is affected. In more extensive cases, degree of corneal scarring (XS) limits visual potential (Figure 10-5).

Figure 10-5. Dry ocular surface with dense stromal scar in a chronic alcoholic. (Reprinted with permission from Dr. Andrew J. Huang.)

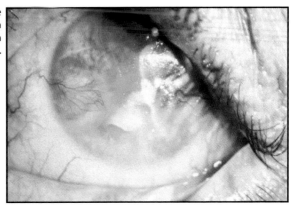

NYCTALOPIA (XN) AND XEROPHTHALMIC FUNDUS (XF)

Night blindness, although not diagnostic of deficiency or a dry eye symptom, can be a useful screening tool in the correct clinical context, as it is the most prevalent form of xerophthalmia. Rhodopsin is dependent on Vitamin A for its regeneration.

Clinical Considerations

- Yellow spots in retinal periphery, outside of vascular arcade.
- Resolves shortly after Vitamin A supplementation, typically within 48 hours.[13]

WORK-UP

I. Careful history to document conditions that typically accompany the clinically obese patient or malnourished patient. Calorie restriction, psychiatric condition, chronic liver disease, and chronic alcohol consumption all contribute to improper absorption and utilization of fat-soluble vitamins. Assess for systemic signs of VAD, such as frequent infections or hyperkeratotic skin. Screen for obstructive sleep apnea, as association with floppy eyelid syndrome may influence management.

II. Slit-lamp examination to evaluate cornea, conjunctiva, eyelid margin, fornices, and tear film with fluorescein.

    A. Schirmer test

      - May show decreased wetting

    B. Tear break-up time

      - Decreased, but may be normal

    C. Vital dyes

- Lissamine green and rose bengal are helpful in detecting conjunctival xerosis; however, they may be quite nonspecific for xerophthalmia

D. Conjunctival impression cytology
   1. Demonstrates loss of goblet cells and keratinization of epithelium
   2. 50% or more abnormal cytology indicates significant risk for deficiency[15]
   3. Can help identify subclinical deficiency[16]
   4. Trachoma/neutrophils on the corneal surface can yield abnormal results

E. Dark adaptation studies and electroretinogram
   - Studies normalize shortly after treatment initiation

F. Corneal culture if superimposed infection suspected
   - Positive culture often yields *Pseudomonas, Pneumococcus, Moraxella*[17]

III. Blood tests and further systemic work-up

A. Serum Vitamin A/retinol
   1. Reference range is 30 to 80 ug/dL
   2. Obtain prior to initiating treatment

B. Serum retinol binding protein
   1. Reference range is 30 to 75 mg/L
   2. Can have ocular symptoms with normal retinol levels and low retinol binding protein

C. Serum zinc levels
   1. Reference range is 75 to 120 ug/d
   2. Zinc deficiency associated with VAD

D. Elucidate underlying cause of deficiency
   1. Check liver enzymes (NASH)
   2. Rule out malabsorption, measles, etc

TREATMENT

General Considerations

- Severe deficiency/keratomalacia should be treated as a medical emergency and prompt more extensive systemic work-up of other common nutritional deficiencies.
- Once VAD has resolved and the ocular surface is stable, consider a corneal transplant if corneal scars limit visual potential.
- Less severe deficiency rapidly responds to Vitamin A treatment (Figure 10-6).

Local Therapy

- Topical Vitamin A, available as retinyl palmitate 0.05%, 4 times/day, has been shown to improve blurred vision.[18] Also useful for persistent Bitot's spots that fail to resolve after systemic therapy.
- Titrate topical Vitamin A to minimum effective dose to limit side effect of irritation.

Figure 10-6. Corneal keratinization in a chronic alcoholic (A) before and (B) after Vitamin A treatment. (Reprinted from *Cornea*, Mannis T, Mannis MJ, Paranjpe DR, Kirkness CM, 676-687, Copyright 2017, with permission from Elsevier.)

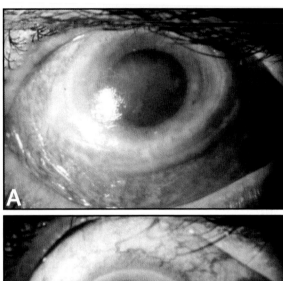

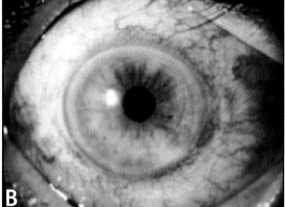

- Lubrication with preservative-free artificial tears and ointment every hour.
- Topical antibiotics for superimposed infection.
- Small perforations (< 2 mm) with little signs of inflammation can be managed with bandage contact lens.

Systemic Therapy

See Table 10-2.

Note

- Vitamin A dosing above the upper limit is not recommended.
- Documented side effects include nausea, vomiting, headache, drowsiness, and hepatotoxicity.

TABLE 10-2

VITAMIN A REPLACEMENT THERAPY	
REFERENCE INTAKE	**ORAL DOSING**
Male	3000 IU PO daily, max: 10,000 IU/day
Female	2330 IU PO daily, max: 10,000 IU/day
Vitamin A deficiency	100,000 IU PO daily for 3 days, then 50,000 IU PO daily for 14 days
Vitamin A deficiency with xerophthalmia	500,000 IU PO daily for 3 days, then 50,000 IU PO daily for 14 days, then 10,000 to 20,000 IU PO daily for 2 months
Prophylaxis, malabsorption syndromes	10,000 to 50,000 IU PO daily
REFERENCE INTAKE	**INTRAMUSCULAR DOSING**
Failed PO therapy, malabsorption	100,000 IU IM daily for 3 days followed by 50,000 IU IM daily for 2 weeks

IM = intramuscularly, IU = international unit, PO = by mouth.

Reprinted with permission from Holland EJ, Mannis MJ, Lee WB. *Ocular Surface Disease: Cornea, Conjunctiva and Tear Film*. London, England: Elsevier/Saunders; 2013:xix, 452.

- Vitamin A toxicity has been associated with increased risk of cardiovascular mortality, lung cancer, and the development of pseudotumor cerebri.[19,20]
- Careful adherence to treatment recommendations in pregnant women.

ESSENTIAL FATTY ACIDS AND CONSIDERATIONS FOR VITAMIN D

Gastric bypass surgery and any state of malnourishment/malabsorption can lead to a plethora of nutritional deficiencies, some of which have been shown clinically and/or in laboratory studies to impact the health of the functional lacrimal unit.

Essential Fatty Acids

It is well known that essential polyunsaturated fatty acids of omega-3 have been useful in the treatment and prevention of dry eye disease. Although no dietary guidelines exist for its use in treating ocular surface disorders, omega-3 fatty acid supplementation has been shown to improve markers of tear film function, decrease markers of ocular surface inflammation, and even demonstrate improvement in ocular surface disease index score.[21,22] It is recommended that patients begin with 1 to 2 g of omega-3 fatty acids/day until reaching a maximum daily dose of 3 g/day.[18] A prior history of gastric bypass surgery magnifies the importance of optimizing essential fatty acid intake.

Vitamin D

One year following gastric bypass surgery, half of all patients will be Vitamin D deficient (VDD). A strong relationship between VDD and chronic inflammation exists. VDD was recently shown to be strongly associated with dry eye disease severity in pre-menopausal women.[23] Furthermore, deficiency in Vitamin D has been found to be a potent instigator of aqueous tear deficiency.[24] Whether these associations are clinically significant in the setting of dry eye disease is yet to be established.

SUMMARY

Signs and symptoms of VDD following gastric bypass surgery mimic those of other ocular surface diseases and can have devastating consequences if left untreated. Clinicians should be aware that this is not a condition only experienced in the developing world, as rates of obesity, malabsorption, and liver disease are on the rise. Prompt recognition of xerophthalmia and initiation of systemic replacement therapy typically leads to resolution of ocular symptoms.

REFERENCES

1. Nguyen NT, Masoomi H, Magno CP, et al. Trends in use of bariatric surgery, 2003-2008. *J Am Coll Surg*. 2011;213(2):261-266.
2. Krachmer JH, Mannis MJ, Holland EJ. *Cornea*. 2nd ed. Philadelphia, PA: Elsevier/Mosby; 2005.
3. Tripathi RC, Tripathi BJ, Raja SC, Partamian LS. Iatrogenic ocular complications in patients after jejunoileal bypass surgery. *Int Surg*. 1993;78(1):68-72.
4. Sommer A. The continuing challenge of vitamin A deficiency. *Ophthalmic Epidemiol*. 2009;16(1):1.
5. Hori Y, Spurr-Michaud SJ, Russo CL, Argueso P, Gipson IK. Effect of retinoic acid on gene expression in human conjunctival epithelium: secretory phospholipase A2 mediates retinoic acid induction of MUC16. *Invest Ophthalmol Vis Sci*. 2005;46(11):4050-4061.
6. Sommer A. Nutritional blindness and xerophthalmia. *Compr Ther*. 1983;9(4):67-71.
7. Sommer A. Conjunctival appearance in corneal xerophthalmia. *Arch Ophthalmol*. 1982;100(6):951-952.
8. Rodger FC, Saiduzzafar H, Grover AD, Fazal A. A reappraisal of the ocular lesion known as Bitot's spot. *Br J Nutr*. 1963;17:475-485.
9. Darby WJ, McGanity WJ, McLaren DS, et al. Bitot's spots and vitamin A deficiency. *Public Health Rep*. 1960;75:738-743.
10. Sommer A. Xerophthalmia, keratomalacia and nutritional blindness. *Int Ophthalmol*. 1990;14(3):195-199.
11. Sommer A, Emran N, Tamba T. Vitamin A-responsive punctate keratopathy in xerophthalmia. *Am J Ophthalmol*. 1979;87(3):330-333.
12. Sommer A, Green WR, Kenyon KR. Clinicohistopathologic correlations in xerophthalmic ulceration and necrosis. *Arch Ophthalmol*. 1982;100(6):953-963.
13. Sommer A. Xerophthalmia and vitamin A status. *Prog Retin Eye Res*. 1998;17(1):9-31.
14. Sommer A. Effects of vitamin A deficiency on the ocular surface. *Ophthalmology*. 1983;90(6):592-600.

15. Carlier C, Coste J, Etchepare M, Amedee-Manesme O. Conjunctival impression cytology with transfer as a field-applicable indicator of vitamin A status for mass screening. *Int J Epidemiol.* 1992;21(2):373-380.

16. Chowdhury S, Kumar R, Ganguly NK, et al. Dynamics of conjunctival impression cytologic changes after vitamin A supplementation. *Br J Nutr.* 1997;77(6):863-869.

17. Valenton MJ, Tan RV. Secondary ocular bacterial infection in hypovitaminosis a xerophthalmia. *Am J Ophthalmol.* 1975;80(4):673-677.

18. Holland EJ, Mannis MJ, Lee WB. *Ocular Surface Disease: Cornea, Conjunctiva and Tear Film.* London, England: Elsevier/Saunders; 2013:xix, 452.

19. Omenn GS, Goodman GE, Thornquist MD, et al. Effects of a combination of beta carotene and vitamin A on lung cancer and cardiovascular disease. *N Engl J Med.* 1996;334(18):1150-1155.

20. Morrice G Jr, Havener WH, Kapetansky F. Vitamin A intoxication as a cause of pseudotumor cerebri. *JAMA.* 1960;173:1802-1805.

21. Brignole-Baudouin F, Baudouin C, Aragona P, et al. A multicentre, double-masked, randomized, controlled trial assessing the effect of oral supplementation of omega-3 and omega-6 fatty acids on a conjunctival inflammatory marker in dry eye patients. *Acta Ophthalmol.* 2011;89(7):e591-e597.

22. Rand AL, Asbell PA. Nutritional supplements for dry eye syndrome. *Curr Opin Ophthalmol.* 2011;22(4):279-282.

23. Yildirim P, Garip Y, Karci AA, Guler T. Dry eye in vitamin D deficiency: more than an incidental association. *Int J Rheum Dis.* 2016;19(1):49-54.

24. Kurtul BE, Ozer PA, Aydinli MS. The association of vitamin D deficiency with tear break-up time and Schirmer testing in non-Sjogren dry eye. *Eye (Lond).* 2015;29(8):1081-1084.

CHAPTER 11

The Patient With Systemic Disease

Albert S. Hazan, MD and Danielle Trief, MD, MSc

KEY POINTS

- Sjögren syndrome (SS), ocular mucous membrane pemphigoid, ocular graft-versus-host disease, thyroid eye disease, diabetes mellitus, and systemic medications play a significant role in causes of dry eye.
- Serologic testing is important in the diagnosis of SS. Anti-Ro/SSA and anti-La/SSB antibodies are present in 58% to 75% of patients with primary SS. Novel biomarkers (Sjögren syndrome testing) are also available for point-of-care testing.
- Anticholinergic drugs such as antidepressants, antipsychotics, antihistamines, and anti-Parkinson's disease contribute to dry eye.
- Dry eye may be the first indication of underlying systemic disease. These patients may require not only topical therapy but also systemic optimization of the disease, requiring a multidisciplinary approach.

The eye is an organ that commonly manifests signs of systemic disease. Ocular manifestations can sometimes be the first indication of a systemic condition and are often part of a constellation of signs characterizing a disorder.

Mah FS, Rhee MK, eds.
Dry Eye Disease: A Practical Guide (pp 109-122).
© 2019 Taylor & Francis Group.

As with any patient, a careful medical history should be performed in patients presenting with dry eye disease. Understanding a patient's systemic disease profile and medication regimen may give insight into the etiology of his or her dry eye. Furthermore, when applicable, treatment may be tailored specifically to the patient's systemic condition.

There are a wide variety of systemic conditions associated with dry eye disease. This chapter focuses on Sjögren syndrome (SS), ocular mucous membrane pemphigoid (OMMP), graft-versus-host disease (GVHD), thyroid eye disease (TED), and diabetes mellitus, as well as the effects of systemic medication on dry eye.

SJÖGREN SYNDROME

SS is a systemic disorder characterized by chronic inflammation of the exocrine glands. The lacrimal and salivary glands are most commonly affected, leading to the classic constellation of aqueous tear deficiency and xerostomia (dry mouth). Exocrine dysfunction at other sites may result in dryness of the skin, nose, throat, trachea, or vagina. SS may be present alone, termed *primary* SS, or it may be associated with other autoimmune diseases (eg, rheumatoid arthritis, systemic lupus erythematosus, scleroderma), which is termed *secondary* SS. Additionally, SS may be associated with other systemic manifestations, including joint, lung, kidney, or liver involvement, termed *extraglandular disease.*

Epidemiology

The incidence of SS is estimated at 1 in 100,000 people, with a higher incidence in Europe and Asia.[1] The female to male predominance is 9:1, with a mean age of diagnosis in the sixth decade of life.[1] In the United States, SS is the second most common rheumatologic disorder behind systemic lupus erythematosus.

Pathophysiology

SS is an autoimmune chronic inflammatory disorder characterized by lymphocytic infiltration of exocrine glands. Aqueous tear deficiency is caused by infiltration of the lacrimal gland by B and CD4 T lymphocytes, which cause cytokine-induced fibrosis and lymphocyte-mediated cell death. Little is understood regarding the etiology of the inflammation, although Epstein-Barr virus and human T-cell lymphotropic virus type 1 have been implicated.[2]

Clinical Manifestations

Patients with SS typically present with symptoms of aqueous tear deficiency and xerostomia, a complex together sometimes referred to as *sicca complex.* As with non-SS, dry eye patients may complain of red eyes, gritty irritation, burning sensation, or photophobia. Exam may reveal conjunctival injection, excessive reflex lacrimation, and corneal and conjunctiva fluorescein or rose bengal staining, predominantly in the inter-palpebral zone. Patients may display salivary or lacrimal gland enlargement.

Diagnosis

Several clinical tests are helpful to properly diagnosis SS, and a comprehensive ophthalmic exam is essential. The ocular surface should be stained with rose bengal, lissamine green, or fluorescein. These ocular dyes stain devitalized epithelial cells. The amount of staining is documented and graded; there are several published scoring systems to aid in diagnosis of SS as well as to monitor progression. The 2 most widely used systems are the van Bijsterveld scoring system and the Sjögren's International Collaborative Clinical Alliance (SICCA) scoring system. Tear break-up time should be noted. A tear break-up time of less than 10 seconds is indicative of rapid evaporation and is common in SS. Schirmer test measures tear production using a filter paper placed in the lower eyelid fornix to assess the extent of wetting of the filter paper. If performed without anesthetic (Schirmer I test), the test measures both basic and reflex tear production. An anesthetized test resulting in less than 5 mm of wetting is indicative of aqueous tear deficiency. Tear osmolarity measurement may also be obtained.

Serologic testing is also important for establishing the diagnosis of SS. Anti-Ro/SSA and anti-La/SSB antibodies are present in 58% to 75% of patients with primary SS. Other autoantibodies may aid in establishing diagnosis as well, including antinuclear antibodies and rheumatoid factor, especially in patients with secondary SS. A new com-mercially available diagnostic test kit (Sjö, Bausch + Lomb) identifies additional bio-markers, including autoantibodies to salivary gland protein-1, parotid secretory protein, and carbonic anhydrase VI, and may allow for earlier diagnosis of SS.

A labial salivary gland biopsy can be obtained to aid in the diagnosis. A classic histo-logical feature of a positive lip biopsy is multiple focal lymphocytic infiltrates. A positive biopsy has a sensitivity of 80%.[3]

There are multiple classification schemes that can be used in the characterization and diagnosis of SS. The 2 most commonly used schemes are the 2002 American-European Consensus Group[3] (AECG) classification criteria and the 2012 SICCA[4] criteria. Both classifications utilize a combination of clinical signs, serologic testing, and histopatho-logical manifestations (Table 11-1). The most recent criteria were published as the 2016 American College of Rheumatology/European League Against Rheumatism,[5] which reflects a collaboration of the AECG and SICCA groups with attention to revising ocular involvement items.

Treatment

The goals of treatment in SS are 2-fold:

1. To provide relief of patient symptoms of ocular irritation, pain, and ocular fatigue
2. To prevent injury to the eye including sterile or infectious keratitis, epithelial ero-sion, neovascularization of the cornea, and ocular surface scarring

For patients with mild disease, management includes a combination of tear replace-ment and environmental modifications. All SS patients should use artificial lubrication

TABLE 11-1A

CRITERIA FOR THE CLASSIFICATION OF SJÖGREN SYNDROME PER THE AMERICAN EUROPEAN CONSENSUS GROUP	
1. OCULAR SYMPTOMS	Daily, persistent, troublesome dry eyes > 3 months OR
	Recurrent sensation of sand/gravel in eyes OR
	Tear substitutes more than 3 times a day
2. ORAL SYMPTOMS	Daily feeling of dry mouth > 3 months OR
	Swollen salivary glands OR
	Drink liquids to assist in swallowing foods
3. OCULAR SIGNS	Schirmer I test > 5 mm in 5 minutes OR
	Rose bengal score > 4 van Bijsterveld score
4. HISTOPATHOLOGICAL FEATURES	Focus score > 1 per 4 mm^2 on minor salivary biopsy
5. SALIVARY GLAND INVOLVEMENT	Delayed uptake or secretion on salivary scintography OR
	Diffuse sialectasis with out obstruction on parotid sialography OR
	Unstimulated salivary flow > 1.5 ml in 15 minutes
6. AUTOANTIBODIES	Antibodies to Ro/SS-A antigens OR
	Antibodies to La/SS-B antigens

Primary Sjögren Syndrome: Presence of 4 out of 6 of the items, or presence of 3 of 4 objective criteria (items 3 through 6)

Secondary Sjögren Syndrome: Well-defined major connective disease and the presence of 1 symptom (items 1 or 2) plus 2 of 3 objective criteria (items 3 through 5)

Exclusion criteria: Preexisting lymphoma, acquired immunodeficiency syndrome, sarcoidosis, chronic GVHD, prior head and neck irradiation, hepatitis C, and use of anticholinergic medications

Adapted from Vitali C, Bombardieri S, Jonsson R, et al. Classification criteria for Sjögren's syndrome: a revised version of the European criteria proposed by the American European Consensus Group. *Ann Rheum Dis.* 2002;61:554-558.

TABLE 11-1B

2016 AMERICAN COLLEGE OF RHEUMATOLOGY/EUROPEAN LEAGUE AGAINST RHEUMATISM CLASSIFICATION CRITERIA FOR PRIMARY SJÖGREN SYNDROME

ITEM	WEIGHTED SCORE
Labial salivary gland with focal lymphocytic sialadenitis and focal score of ≥1 foci/4 mm^2	3
Anti-SS-A/Ro positive	3
Ocular Staining Score ≥5 or van Bijsterveld score ≥4	1
Schirmer test ≤5 mm/5 min in at least 1 eye	1
Unstimulated whole saliva flow rate ≤0.1 mL/min	1

A score of ≥4 signifies primary SS.

Exclusion criteria: History of head and neck radiation, active hepatitis C virus infection, AIDS, sarcoidosis, amyloidosis, GVHD, IgG4-related disease

Adapted from Shiboski CH, Shiboski SC, Seror R, et al. 2016 American College of Rheumatology/ European League Against Rheumatism classification criteria for primary Sjögren's syndrome: a consensus and data-driven methodology involving three international patient cohorts. *Ann Rheum Dis.* 2017;76:9-16.

as needed and a longer-acting lubricating ointment may be useful at night.[6] Education should involve avoidance of dry ambient environments, avoidance of medications that exacerbate drying of the ocular surface, and attention to eyelid exposure. Moisture-conserving eyewear, such as side shields or goggles, have been developed and may be helpful, especially in low humidity environments.[6]

Patients who have moderate disease and no significant improvement with artificial tears can be treated with topical cyclosporine A (starting dose 0.05% 1 drop twice a day), a powerful suppressor of T-cell function.[7] More recently approved by the US Food and Drug Administration, topical lifitegrast 5% (1 drop twice a day) is a lymphocyte function-associated antigen-1 antagonist available for treatment of dry eye. Punctal occlusion may also be beneficial and can be permanent or temporary. Typically, temporary occlusion, such as collagen punctal plugs, are initiated. If there is symptomatic relief, permanent occlusion with thermal cautery may be considered.

Severe disease typically requires more aggressive and often systemic treatment, usually in patients with systemic and extraglandular disease. Hydroxychloroquine (6 to 7 mg/kg/day for 24 to 48 months) has shown improvement in symptoms and objective testing of dry eye in 50% to 60% of SS patients.[8] Rituximab has shown evidence of benefit for extraglandular manifestations, though less promising for dry eye and dry mouth symptoms. Autologous tears, a dilution of a patient's serum compounded as eye drops, have also been shown to be of benefit for dry eye symptoms in refractory cases.[9]

Additionally, large diameter gas-permeable contact lenses may be used for select cases. The contact lens maintains a fluid reservoir anterior to the corneal epithelium.

Ocular Mucous Membrane Pemphigoid

OMMP, formerly known as *ocular cicatricial pemphigoid*, is a heterogeneous group of chronic inflammatory disorders that cause blistering of the mucous membranes around the body. OMMP can affect the mucosa of the eyes, pharynx, larynx, genitals, and anus. Approximately 80% of patients with OMMP have ocular involvement.[10]

Epidemiology

The incidence of OMMP is between 1 in 8000 and 1 in 46,000 patients. Reports suggest a female predominance with typical age of diagnosis in the seventh decade of life.[10] Only a handful of cases have been reported in infants, children, and adolescents, and treatment responses in these patient groups do not differ greatly from those in adults. There is no known geographic or racial predilection.[11]

Pathophysiology

Although the exact mechanism of OMMP is unknown, it is thought to be a cytotoxic (type II) hypersensitivity. Cell damage occurs as a result of aberrant production of autoantibodies directed against normal cell surface antigens of the mucuosal epithelial basement membrane zone. There are several basement membrane antigen targets implicated in OMMP, including bullous pemphigoid antigen II (BP180), laminin 5, $\alpha6\beta4$ integrin, and others.[11] Binding of autoantibodies to these antigens stimulates an inflammatory cascade involving the secretion of cytokines and recruitment of inflammatory cells. These inflammatory cells in turn release profibrotic cytokines such as transforming growth factor (TGF-β) and interferon (INF-γ), which lead to the clinical manifestations of OMMP.

Certain mutations in HLA-DR4 and HLA-DR5 have been shown to be associated with OMMP; however, not all patients with OMMP will have these mutations, limiting the usefulness of genetic testing in suspected patients.[12]

Clinical Manifestations

OMMP is characterized by a chronic cicatrizing conjunctivitis whose clinical manifestations depend on the stage of disease. It is a bilateral disease but may be asymmetric. Often it develops unilaterally followed by involvement of the fellow eye several years later.[13]

Early disease presents with signs and symptoms of chronic or relapsing conjunctivitis. Patients may complain of tearing, irritation, burning, and mucous discharge. Exam may be significant for conjunctival hyperemia, edema, ulceration, and tear dysfunction. Frank bullae are rarely seen. As the disease progresses, conjunctival subepithelial fibrosis appears. The fibrosis begins as fine grey-white linear opacities. As the fibrosis continues, conjunctival shrinking occurs and symblepharon formation occurs. Symblepharon, defined as fibrotic adhesions between bulbar and palpebral conjunctiva, typically begin in the inferior fornix. An inferior forniceal depth of less than 8 mm is abnormal and indicative of symblepharon. Recurrent attacks of conjunctival inflammation can lead to destruction of goblet cells and eventually obstruction of the lacrimal gland ductules. The resultant aqueous and mucous tear deficiency leads to further keratinization of an already-thickened and abnormal conjunctiva. Severe scarring and fibrosis can lead to ankyloblepharon (fusion of the upper and lower eyelid margin), entropion (inward turning of the eyelid margins), and trichiasis (inward growth of eyelashes), all which leads to recurrent corneal epithelial defects, neovascularization, ulceration, and scarring. Additionally, conjunctival scarring may lead to impairment in extraocular movements and lagophthalmos.[13]

In 1986, Foster proposed a clinical staging system to assist in assessment of disease severity and response to treatment (Table 11-2).[13]

Diagnosis

Pathological specimen of involved tissue can be obtained to support the diagnosis. In patients with extraocular lesions, such as skin or oral mucosa, a biopsy from these sites may be easily obtained. If only conjunctival involvement is present, a conjunctival biopsy should be obtained.[14] All specimens should be evaluated with direct immunofluorescence and thus require proper tissue handling with an immunoperoxidase assay. Characteristic findings include linear deposits of IgG, IgA, or C3 of the basement membrane zone of the conjunctiva.

Differential Diagnosis

The differential diagnosis of OMMP includes any cause of cicatrizing conjunctivitis. Postinfectious conjunctivitis, autoimmune conditions such as sarcoidosis, scleroderma, lichen planus, Stevens-Johnson syndrome, dermatitis herpetiformis, epidermolysis bullosa, atopic blepharoconjunctivitis, GVHD, and prior conjunctival trauma can all present with similar conjunctival scarring. Definitive diagnosis can be made on histopathology as above.

Treatment

A multidisciplinary approach is often necessary to adequately manage patients with this systemic multisystem disease. The goal of ocular treatment is to prevent conjunctival and corneal scarring. Nonpharmacologic therapy with ocular lubrication, proper eyelid hygiene with eyelid scrubs and warm compresses, and epilation of eyelashes for trichiasis should all be employed when appropriate. In mild disease, first-line treatment is dapsone (50 to 200 mg/day for 12 weeks). Dapsone is a sulfonamide antibiotic with anti-inflammatory properties. It has been proven effective in OMMP by decreasing inflammation through its inhibition of myeloperoxidase, an enzyme important in neutrophil-mediated oxidative inflammation.[14] It is important that patients be screened for

TABLE 11-2

CLINICAL STAGING SYSTEM FOR OCULAR MUCOUS MEMBRANE PEMPHIGOID	
STAGE I	Presence of chronic conjunctivitis with subepithelial fibrosis, best seen as white bands in the upper and lower tarsal conjunctiva
STAGE II	Inferior forniceal foreshortening
STAGE III	Appearance of symblepharon
STAGE IV	End stage disease, characterized by ankyloblepharon, severe sicca syndrome, and extreme ocular surface keratinization
Adapted from Foster CS. Cicatricial pemphigoid. *Trans Am Ophthalmol Soc.* 1986;84:527-663.	

glucose 6-phosphate dehydrogenase (G6PD) deficiency if dapsone therapy is considered; hemolytic anemia can occur in patients with G6PD deficiency. Other immunosuppressive agents can be used including methotrexate (5 to 25 mg/week), mycophenolate mofetil (500 to 1000 mg twice daily), and azathioprine (50 to 125 mg/day).[15] Severe disease may require more aggressive treatment to minimize scarring and prevent visual loss. A combination of cyclophosphamide (2 mg/kg/day) and prednisone (1 mg/kg/day) has been found to be very effective for severe OMMP.[14]

Newer research has also shown that intravenous immunoglobulin may be effective in refractory cases.[16] Lastly, early data for rituximab infusion (375 mg/m[2]) once weekly for 4 weeks for 1 or 2 cycles, has shown promise for treatment in severe OMMP.[17] While surgical intervention may be required in certain situations, it will increase ocular inflammation and thus patients should be pretreated with immunomodulatory drugs to promote optimal surgical outcomes. Surgical interventions include repair of symblepharon when affecting eyelid function, eyelid deformity repair, amniotic membrane transplant, limbal stem cell transplant, or corneal transplant, when clinically indicated.

OCULAR GRAFT-VERSUS-HOST DISEASE

Ocular GVHD is a complication of allogeneic hematological stem cell transplant. Acute systemic GVHD develops in approximately 40% of human leukocyte antigen–matched patients. Chronic GVHD develops in 30% to 70% of transplanted patients.[18] Acute systemic GVHD occurs in the first 100 days post transplant and is characterized by dermatitis, hepatitis, and enteritis. By contrast, chronic GVHD occurs 100 days or more post transplant. Features of chronic GVHD include obstructive pulmonary disease, oral ulcers, ocular GVHD, and neuromuscular disease (myasthenia gravis–like symptoms or polymyositis). Ocular GVHD occurs in 60% to 90% of patients with chronic GVHD.[18]

Pathophysiology

GVHD is a T cell–mediated process initiated when donor lymphocytes interact with host histocompatibility antigens. This leads to an inflammatory cascade involving cellular mediators and the activation of cytotoxic T lymphocytes, natural killer cells, and soluble inflammatory agents such as tumor necrosis factor-alpha, INF-γ, interleukin-1, and nitric oxide.[18] In the eye, this inflammatory cascade leads to infiltration and fibrosis of the lacrimal gland, decreased density in conjunctival goblet cells, and conjunctival scarring.

Clinical Manifestations

In acute GVHD, ocular disease typically consists of conjunctival hyperemia, chemosis, and pseudomembrane formation. Chronic GVHD is characterized by dry eye (aqueous deficiency and evaporative dysfunction) and chronic blepharitis. This process may lead to conjunctival scarring as well as corneal manifestations, such as punctate keratopathy, filamentary keratitis, and painful erosions. With breakdown of the corneal surface, secondary corneal infections and even perforations are possible.

Treatment

Systemic treatment for GVHD is important, but ocular manifestations usually require additional topical therapy. Patients should be treated with aggressive topical lubrication including preservative-free artificial tears. The addition of topical anti-inflammatory medications may be required such as topical steroids or topical cyclosporine A. Topical cyclosporine A (0.5% or 1% twice daily) is a T-cell inhibitor, which can downregulate inflammatory cytokines in the conjunctiva and lacrimal gland. It has been shown that when used 1 month prior to bone marrow transplant, topical cyclosporine A significantly reduces ocular symptoms of GVHD compared to those who were not pretreated.[19] Other treatments include punctal plugs, autologous serum tears, and therapeutic contact lenses, including the BostonSight Prosthetic Replacement of the Ocular Surface Ecosystem (PROSE).[20]

THYROID EYE DISEASE

TED is an inflammatory orbitopathy in the setting of systemic autoimmune thyroid disease. The classic findings of TED include eyelid retraction, lagophthalmos, exophthalmos, dysmotility, and diplopia.

Epidemiology

The overall incidence of TED is 16 women and 3 men per 100,000 per year. Approximately 20% to 25% of patients with Graves' disease have some level of TED.[21]

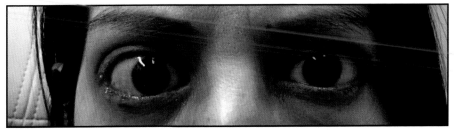

Figure 11-1. Patient with TED. Note the eyelid retraction, relative proptosis, and scleral show of the right eye.

Pathophysiology

The pathogenesis of TED involves activation of orbital fibroblasts, which contain a higher number of thyroid-stimulating receptor (TSH-R) and insulin-like growth factor-1 receptor (IGF-1R) than other fibroblasts. Stimulation of these receptors in TED leads to a complex inflammatory cascade involving B- and T-cell activation and cytokine release, which, in turn, results in an upregulation and production of glycosaminoglycans and adipogenesis in the extraocular muscles and orbit. This activation leads to an increase in the volume of the extraocular muscles and retro-orbital connective tissue, which, in turn, causes proptosis, strabismus, and venous congestion (Figure 11-1).[22]

Clinical Manifestations

Notably, 3.9% of dry eye patients suffer from TED, much higher than the annual incidence of 0.2% for TED in the general population.[23] Similarly, in a cohort study of 60 patients with TED, 97% suffered from dry eye symptomatology.[24] The dry eye symptoms in patients with TED are attributable to ocular inflammation rather than aqueous tear deficiency, as most patients with TED have normal tear break-up time and Schirmer tests.[23] Interestingly, there has been no correlation with dry eye symptomatology and eyelid retraction or proptosis. Instead, the orbital inflammation is thought to lead to conjunctival injection, episcleral inflammation, and chemosis specifically over the extraocular muscles, causing the dry eye symptomatology.[23]

Treatment

Treatment for active TED may involve systemic corticosteroids, orbital radiation, and in severe cases (causing optic neuropathy) surgical decompression. Treatment of dry eye symptoms in TED is often with topical anti-inflammatories such as topical steroids or topical cyclosporine A (0.5% to 1% twice daily) given its inflammatory etiology. Additionally, warm compresses, artificial tears, and punctal plugs can be used. This treatment strategy has shown improvement in 72% of TED patients with dry eye.[21]

DIABETES MELLITUS AND DRY EYE

Epidemiology

Diabetes mellitus is a leading cause of visual impairment in the 20- to 74-year age group, due to retinopathy and cataract.[25] It has been shown that dry eye is another complicating ocular condition for diabetes mellitus patients, with a prevalence of 15% to 33% in those over 65 years old.[26]

Pathophysiology

The mechanism in which diabetes causes dry eye remains unclear but is likely a combination of neuropathy, metabolic dysfunction, and abnormal lacrimal secretions.[26,27] A tear break-up time value lower than 10 seconds (abnormal) was found in 94.2% of diabetes mellitus patients.[27] A direct correlation was shown between the glycated hemoglobin (HbA1C) and the presence of dry eye syndrome.[28] Additionally, there has been an association between diabetic retinopathy and dry eye syndrome.[29] It has been shown that people with diabetes have both a decreased basal tear secretion, thought to be due to peripheral neuropathy affecting lacrimal gland function, as well as decreased reflex tear secretion, due to corneal neuropathy and decreased cornea sensitivity.[30]

Clinical Manifestations

Clinical presentation is similar to patients presenting with aqueous tear deficiency in the absence of diabetes mellitus. Patients complain of a gritty sensation, decreased visual acuity, and photophobia. Additionally, on exam, decreased goblet cell density can be seen and corneal sensitivity may be reduced. Complications of diabetes mellitus–related dry eye include superficial punctate keratopathy, trophic ulceration, and persistent epithelial defects, due to poor wound healing.

Treatment

The approach to treating dry eye in patients with diabetes is similar to the treatment of patients with aqueous tear deficiency and includes topical lubrication, punctal occlusion, and autologous serum tears. Occasionally, patients with diabetes will develop a neurotrophic cornea, and a bandage contact lens can be used in the short term for persistent epithelial defects. A multidisciplinary coordination of care must be taken to optimize blood sugar control and systemic comorbidities of diabetes mellitus.

SYSTEMIC MEDICATIONS AND DRY EYE

The incidence of dry eye is significantly greater in those taking chronic medications. Given the relative high vascularity of the conjunctiva and lacrimal gland, these structures are subject to high penetration rates of drugs absorbed into the systemic circulation.[31]

Many of the systemic drugs known to cause dry eye have anticholinergic action. Anticholinergic drugs are postulated to affect the aqueous and mucous secretions.[31] Antidepressant, antipsychotic, anti-Parkinson's disease, and antihistamine drugs are all known to have anticholinergic action and thus can contribute to dry eye symptoms. Additionally, sex hormones, particularly androgens, greatly influence lacrimal and meibomian secretions leading to dry eye symptoms.[32] Other systemic medications such as certain chemotherapeutic drugs (busulfan, methotrexate, and mitomycin C), antihypertensives (beta blockers and angiotensin-converting enzyme inhibitors), acne medication (isotretinoin), and antiarrhythmics can cause dry eye symptoms for unknown reasons.[31]

When approaching a patient with dry eye, it is essential to perform a thorough review of a patient's systemic medications, as these medications may be contributing to his or her dry eye disease. Treatment involves coordination of care with medical doctors. Options include cessation of the offending medication if deemed safe, switching to another medication, or switching to topical therapy (eg, acne medication). Often a patient needs to stay on the systemic medication for optimal health. In these situations, the patient should be made aware of the side effects of the medication, and his or her concomitant dry eye can be treated accordingly.

SUMMARY

There are various systemic diseases that can lead to or exacerbate dry eye disease. The mechanism of dry eye in these patients depends on the particular systemic disease and includes chronic inflammation, decreased corneal sensitivity, decreased basal and reflex tear production, and eyelid malposition. Successful treatment of dry eye disease in these patients requires not only local therapy but optimal control of their systemic disease. Due to the complexities of managing patients with multi-organ disease, it is imperative to employ a multidisciplinary approach in the care of these patients.

REFERENCES

1. Qin B, Wang J, Yang Z, et al. Epidemiology of primary Sjögren's syndrome: a systematic review and meta analysis. *Ann Rheum Dis*. 2015;74:1983-1989.
2. Nishioka K. HTLV-I arthropathy and Sjögren syndrome. *J Acquir Immune Defic Syndr Hum Retrovirol*. 1996;13(Suppl 1):S57-S62.
3. Vitali C, Bombardieri S, Jonsson R, et al. Classification criteria for Sjögren's syndrome: a revised version of the European criteria proposed by the American European Consensus Group. *Ann Rheum Dis*. 2002;61:554-558.

4. Shiboski SC, Shiboski CH, Criswell LA, et al. American College of Rheumatology classification criteria for Sjogren's syndrome: a data-driven expert consensus approach in the Sjogren's International Collaborative Clinical Alliance Cohort. *Arthritis Care Res.* 2012;64:475-487.

5. Shiboski CH, Shiboski SC, Seror R, et al. 2016 American College of Rheumatology/European League Against Rheumatism classification criteria for primary Sjögren's syndrome: a consensus and data-driven methodology involving three international patient cohorts. *Ann Rheum Dis.* 2017;76:9-16.

6. Akpek EK, Lindsley KB, Adyanthaya RS, et al. Treatment of Sjögren's syndrome associated dry eye an evidence-based review. *Ophthalmology* 2011;118:1242-1252.

7. Ramos-Casals M, Tzioufas AG, Stone JH, et al. Treatment of primary Sjögren syndrome: a systematic review. *JAMA.* 2010;304:452-460.

8. Fox RI, Dixon R, Guarrasi V, Krubel S. Treatment of primary Sjögren's syndrome with hydroxychloroquine: a retrospective, open-label study. *Lupus.* 1996;5(Suppl 1):S31-S36.

9. Yoon KC, Heo H, Im SK, et al. Comparison of autologous serum and umbilical cord serum eye drops for dry eye syndrome. *Am J Ophthalmol.* 2007;144:86-92.

10. Broussard KC, Leung TG, Moradi A, Thorne JE, Fine JD. Autoimmune bullous diseases with skin and eye involvement: cicatricial pemphigoid, pemphigus vulgaris, and pemphigus paraneoplastica. *Clin Dermatol.* 2016;34(2):205-213.

11. Schmidt E, Zillikens D. Pemphigoid diseases. *Lancet.* 2013;381:320-332.

12. Ahmed R, Foster S, Zaltas M, et al. Association of DQw7 (DQB1*0301) with ocular cicatricial pemphigoid. *Proc Natl Acad Sci U S A.* 1991;88:11579-11582.

13. Foster CS. Cicatricial pemphigoid. *Trans Am Ophthalmol Soc.* 1986;84:527-663.

14. Chan LS, Ahmed AR, Anhalt GJ, et al. The first international consensus on mucous membrane pemphigoid: definition, diagnostic criteria, pathogenic factors, medical treatment, and prognostic indicators. *Arch Dermatol.* 2002;138:370-379.

15. Saw VP, Dart JK, Rauz S, et al. Immunosuppressive therapy for ocular mucous membrane pemphigoid strategies and outcomes. *Ophthalmology.* 2008;115:253-261.

16. Foster CS, Ahmed AR. Intravenous immunoglobulin therapy for ocular cicatricial pemphigoid: a preliminary study. *Ophthalmology.* 1999;106:2136-2143.

17. Le Roux-Villet C, Prost-Squarcioni C, Alexandre M, et al. Rituximab for patients with refractory mucous membrane pemphigoid. *Arch Dermatol.* 2011;147:843-849.

18. Hessen M, Akpek EK. Ocular graft-versus-host disease. *Curr Opin Allergy Clin Immunol.* 2012;12(5):540-547.

19. 1Malta JB, Soong HK, Shtein RM, et al. Treatment of ocular graft-versus-host disease with topical cyclosporine 0.05%. *Cornea.* 2010;29(12):1392-1396.

20. Townley JR, Dana R, Jacobs DS. Keratoconjunctivitis sicca manifestations in ocular graft versus host disease: pathogenesis, presentation, prevention, and treatment. *Semin Ophthalmol.* 2011;26(4-5):251-260.

21. Bartley GB, Fatourechi V, Kadrmas EF, et al. Clinical features of Graves' ophthalmopathy in an incidence cohort. *Am J Ophthalmology.* 1996;121:284-290.

22. Durairaj VD. Clinical perspectives of thyroid eye disease. *Am J Med.* 2006;119:1027-1028.

23. Gupta A, Sadeghi PB, Akpek EK. Occult thyroid eye disease in patients presenting with dry eye symptoms. *Am J Ophthalmol.* 2009;147(5):919-923.

24. Coulter I, Frewin S, Krassas GE, et al. Psychological implications of Graves' orbitopathy. *Eur J Endocrinol.* 2007;157:127-131.

25. Harrison TR. Diabetes mellitus. In: Braunwald E, Fauci AS, Kasper DL, Hauser SL, Longo DL, Jameson JL, eds. Harrison's Principles of Internal Medicine 15th ed. New York, NY: McGraw-Hill; 2001:2121.

26. Manaviat MR, Rashidi M, Afkhami-Ardekani M. Prevalence of dry eye syndrome and diabetic retinopathy in type 2 diabetic patients. *BMC Ophthalmology.* 2008;8:10.

27. Inoue K, Kato S, Ohara C, Numaga J, Amanto S, Oshika T. Ocular and systemic factors relevant to diabetic keratoepitheliopathy. *Cornea.* 2001;20(8):798-801.

28. Seifart U, Strempel I. The dry eye syndrome and diabetes mellitus. *Ophthalmologe.* 1994;91(2):235-239.

29. Nepp J, Abela C, Polzer I, Derbolav A, Wedrich A. Is there a correlation between the severity of diabetic retinopathy and keratoconjunctivitis sicca? *Cornea.* 2000;19(4):487-491.

30. Cousen P, Cackett P, Bennett H, Swa K, Dhillon B. Tear production and corneal sensitivity in diabetes. *J Diabetes Complications.* 2007;21(6):371-373.

31. Wong J, Lan W, Ong LM, Tong L. Non-hormonal systemic medications and dry eye. *Ocul Surf.* 2011;9(4):212-226.

32. Creuzot-Garcher C. Ocular dryness related to systemic medications. *J Fr Ophtalmol.* 2009;32:64-70.

CHAPTER 12

The Patient With Other Ocular Disease

Frank X. Cao, MD; Nataliya Pokeza, MD; Allison Rizzuti, MD; and
Stephen C. Kaufman, MD, PhD

KEY POINTS

- Aniridia is a rare, congenital, panocular disease caused by a PAX6 gene mutation. Dry eye and limbal stem cell dysfunction can be diagnosed in the majority of these patients.
- Superior limbic keratoconjunctivitis is an inflammatory disorder of the superior bulbar and upper palpebral conjunctiva with an associated superior superficial keratitis. It is linked with keratoconjunctivitis sicca, hypothyroidism, and hypoparathyroidism.
- Ocular allergy affects about 20% to 40% of the US population, with seasonal/perennial allergic conjunctivitis being the most prevalent form.
- Herpes simplex virus and herpes zoster virus may damage the ophthalmic division of the fifth cranial nerve, leading to diminished corneal sensation and resultant neurotrophic keratopathy.
- Amniotic membrane and limbal stem cell transplantation may be helpful in aniridia and alkali injury.

Mah FS, Rhee MK, eds.
Dry Eye Disease: A Practical Guide (pp 123-132).
© 2019 Taylor & Francis Group.

Dry eyes are almost always the result of some underlying abnormality. It is imperative that the clinician identify the underlying etiology of a patient's dry eyes. A part of any initial management should address the cause; no matter whether the dry eyes are the result of a systemic disease, local ocular disease, or trauma.

It is particularly important that the clinician be aware of other etiologies of dry eyes. Uncommon causes of dry eye, such as lymphoma, graft-versus-host disease and HIV should always be considered because the lacrimal gland, accessory lacrimal glands, and mucous membranes are frequently affected by inflammatory disorders as well as antigen antibody reactions, which will be discussed elsewhere.[1,2] However, dry eyes, as the result of other ocular disorders, also require the recognition and treatment of the underlying disorder and their sequella.

ANIRIDIA AND DRY EYE

Aniridia is a rare congenital bilateral apoplasia of the iris caused by a PAX6 gene mutation that affects 1 in 100,000 births.[3-5] A panocular disorder, aniridia affects the cornea, anterior chamber, lens, and retina. The majority of cases are familial and sporadic aniridia may be associated with Wilms tumor.[4,5] Clinical features include photophobia, nystagmus, cataracts, glaucoma, strabismus, amblyopia, and reduced visual acuity (20/100 to 20/200 range).[5]

Dry eye with diminished tear production and instability of the tear film is reported in up to 95% of aniridia patients. While there are reports of normal Schirmer test results in aniridia eyes, the majority of patients have reduced tear break-up time, decreased tear meniscus level, conjunctival mucinous hyperplasia, positive fluorescein and rose bengal corneal, and conjunctival staining, as well as stenosis of meibomian orifices. Limbal stem cell dysfunction and/or deficiency can be diagnosed in up to 100% of aniridia eyes. Presence of various degrees of aniridic keratopathy with corneal pannus, recurrent erosions and progressive corneal opacification and vascularization is reported in all patients with aniridia. The extent of dry eye correlates with the severity of keratopathy.[4,5]

Evaluation of the quality of tear film, the 3 layers of tears and their producing cells are important in the management of dryness in aniridia eyes. Early treatment modalities include lubricants, nonsteroidal and steroidal anti-inflammatory medications that could interrupt the inflammatory cascade and delay corneal changes.[6] Autologous serum tears are rich in growth factors and have been shown to improve mild and moderate degrees of aniridic keratopathy.[7] Amniotic membrane and stem cell transplantation may be necessary in patients with severe corneal changes and limbal stem cell deficiency (LCSD).[5,8]

THYROID EYE DISEASE AND DRY EYE

Thyroid-associated ophthalmopathy (TAO) is an autoimmune disorder caused by retro-orbital inflammation and is generally associated with Graves' disease and rarely with Hashimoto's thyroiditis.[9] Characteristic features include eyelid retraction,

TABLE 12-1

NOSPECS CLASSIFICATION SYSTEM FOR GRAVES' OPHTHALMOPATHY

CLASS 0	No signs or symptoms
CLASS 1	Only signs (limited to upper eyelid retraction and stare, with or without eyelid lag)
CLASS 2	Soft tissue involvement (edema of conjunctiva and eyelids, conjunctival injection)
CLASS 3	Proptosis
CLASS 4	Extraocular muscle involvement (usually with diplopia)
CLASS 5	Corneal involvement (primarily due to lagophthalmos)
CLASS 6	Sight loss (due to optic nerve involvement)

proptosis, eyelid lag, periorbital edema, optic neuropathy, restrictive ocular myopathy and ocular surface disorders (Table 12-1). Dry eye has been reported in up to 85% of TAO patients and is the most frequent cause of ocular discomfort.[9-11]

Increased ocular surface exposure and inadequate blinking due to proptosis and eyelid retraction result in poor tear film distribution over the ocular surface and allow for excess tear evaporation (Figure 12-1).[9,12] Reduced aqueous tear production may result from inflammatory processes within the lacrimal gland which has been shown to express thyroid-stimulating hormone receptors that could function as a potential target for the autoantibodies in Graves' disease.[13] Patients have shorter tear film break-up time, tear film instability, and significant corneal and conjunctival damage as seen with rose bengal and fluorescein staining. Elevated tear film osmolarity in TAO patients has been reported to stimulate the production of proinflammatory markers such as tumor necrosis factor-α (TNF-α) and matrix metalloproteinase-9 (MMP-9) that may lead to ocular damage and dry eye.[9,10]

While the treatment should be aimed at managing the underlying thyroid disorder, orbital radiotherapy may contribute to the development or progression of dry eye. In addition to daytime lubrication, overnight lubricant therapy, moisture chamber goggles and eyelid taping may be necessary to treat the dry eye from lagophthalmos. Surgical management of proptosis and dysfunctional eyelid position, such as orbital decompression and tarsorrhaphy, can help protect the ocular surface. Anti-inflammatory agents such as topical cyclosporine A and steroids, as well as tetracyclines, have been found beneficial in treatment of dry eye in TAO patients.[9,12]

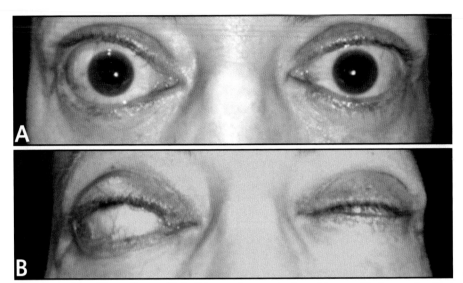

Figure 12-1. Thyroid eye disease. (A) Eyelid retraction, proptosis, and temporal bulbar conjunctival injection noted bilaterally. (B) Bilateral conjunctival and right inferior corneal exposure on attempted eyelid closure in setting of TAO. (Reprinted with permission from Roman Shinder, MD.)

SUPERIOR LIMBIC KERATOCONJUNCTIVITIS

Superior limbic keratoconjuntivitis (SLK) is an inflammatory disorder of the superior bulbar and upper palpebral conjunctiva with associated superior superficial keratitis. SLK is a chronic condition, which frequently takes a relapsing and remitting course, leading to epidermalization and kertinization or pannus of the superior conjunctiva and cornea. In severe long-standing cases, LCSD can result.

The condition is bilateral but can be asymmetric, and affects women more than men. Patients with SLK complain of burning, redness, and other non-specific dry eye-like symptoms, but on physical exam display a distinct triad of signs, which include; papillary reaction of the superior palpebral conjunctiva, sectoral hyperemia of the superior bulbar conjunctiva, and superior superficial punctate keratoconjuntivitis (Table 12-2 and Figure 12-2). The superior conjunctiva will often appear thickened and redundant. Rose bengal dye will demonstrate coarse punctate staining.

SLK is associated with keratoconjunctivitis sicca, hypothyroidism and hypoparathyroidism, which suggests an autoimmune etiology. While the pathogenesis remains unclear, it is thought that mechanical friction between the upper palpebral and bulbar conjunctiva leads to a blink-related microtrauma and the development of SLK in susceptible individuals.[14]

Various treatment options have been attempted with variable results, including 0.5% silver nitrate, artificial tear drops, topical corticosteroids, autologous serum tears, cyclosporine A, punctal plugs, and bandage contact lenses. Conjunctival resection with or without amniotic membrane graft is an effective technique for patients not responsive

TABLE 12-2

SUPERIOR LIMBIC KERATOCONJUNCTIVITIS SIGNS
Papillary reaction of the superior palpebral conjunctiva
Hyperemia of superior bulbar conjunctiva
Superficial punctate keratoconjunctivitis

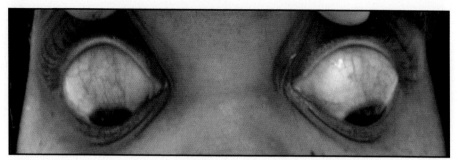

Figure 12-2. Superior limbic keratoconjunctivitis in a patient with hypothyroidism.

to medical therapies.[15] Injection of botulinum toxin into the muscle of Riolan has been proposed to be an effective alternative.[16] With so many alternative treatments, it should be evident that there is no single solution that is effective 100% of the time.

DRY EYE AND OCULAR ALLERGY

Allergic conjunctivitis is a common inflammatory disorder of the ocular surface that may accompany systemic disease. Ocular allergies affect approximately 20% to 40% of the US population, with seasonal/perennial allergic conjunctivitis being the most prevalent form.[17] Differentiating between dry eye disease and seasonal or perennial allergic conjunctivitis can sometimes be challenging (Table 12-3), as both conditions may present with non-specific symptoms such as redness and irritation. In addition, it is not uncommon for patients to have both disorders with one condition exacerbating the signs and symptoms of the other.[18] Vernal keratoconjunctivitis, atopic keratoconjunctivitis, and drug-induced dermatoconjunctivitis are less common forms of ocular allergy that are more easily distinguished from dry eye syndrome due to their specific presentations and clinical signs.

The clinical history is critical in allergic eye disease, as it frequently will guide the clinician to the offending allergen. Patients with seasonal allergic conjunctivitis experience symptoms during specific times of the year when environmental allergen counts such as pollen or ragweed are highest. Perennial allergic conjunctivitis to allergens such as dust, mold, and animals may occur year round. Itching is the predominant symptom in ocular allergy and it often will differentiate allergic disease from the burning sensation

TABLE 12-3

DRY EYE DISEASE VERSUS ALLERGIC CONJUNCTIVITIS

	DRY EYE DISEASE	ALLERGIC CONJUNCTIVITIS
AGE GROUP	Female > Male Increased prevalence with age	Common in pediatric age group Male > Female in vernal keratoconjunctivitis
MEDICAL HISTORY	Systemic disease (hypothyroid, Sjögren syndrome)	Exposure to known allergen Systemic atopy (eczema, rhinitis, asthma)
SEASONALITY	Worse in cold/dry seasons	Worse during seasons with high pollen count
SYMPTOMS	Burning Foreign body sensation Tearing Photophobia	Itching Photophobia Tearing
SIGNS	Decreased tear break-up time Mild injection Punctate keratopathy	Conjunctival papillary reaction Mild to moderate injection Watery discharge Eyelid edema Chemosis

of dry eye syndrome. Redness, tearing and foreign body sensation are common complaints in both disorders. On physical exam, patients with allergic conjunctivitis display conjunctival hyperemia and papillae, and in more severe cases, eyelid edema, chemosis, and a watery discharge.

Avoidance of environmental allergens is recommended for patients with ocular allergy, but is usually not feasible, particularly in cases of seasonal allergic conjunctivitis. Topical antihistamine drops and/or mast cell stabilizers are the mainstay of therapy and have been shown to be superior to systemic therapy which can have a significant drying effect on the ocular surface.[19] Artificial tears may also be beneficial in 2 ways: 1) it washes allergens from the ocular surface; and 2) the drops can be kept in a refrigerator, which adds the benefit of decreasing histamine release and other inflammatory effects by cooling the ocular surface.

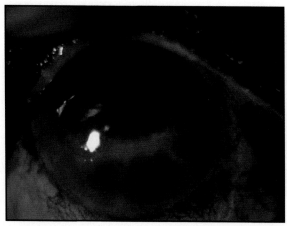

Figure 12-3. An HSV dendrite, which may lead to corneal neuropathy. Check corneal sensation for evidence of a neurotrophic cornea.

NEUROTROPHIC HSV/HZV–RELATED DRY EYE

Herpes simplex virus (HSV) and Herpes zoster virus (HZ) are ubiquitous DNA viruses. HSV establishes latency in the trigeminal ganglion following primary infection of the facial region, where it may undergo reactivation. HZ results from neuronal reactivation of latent varicella zoster virus (VZV), a contagious childhood illness with characteristic vesicular skin lesions. Herpes zoster ophthalmicus (HZO) is defined when HZ involves the ophthalmic division of the fifth cranial nerve. HSV and HZO may damage nerves and result in diminished corneal sensation, which results in a neurotrophic keratopathy with tear dysfunction, loss of goblet cells, and epithelial breakdown (Figure 12-3).[20-26]

Treatment of neurotrophic keratopathy related dry eye should focus on promoting epithelial healing and prevention of further epithelial breakdown. If possible, topical and systemic medications that can worsen dryness or neuropathy should be discontinued. Application of frequent preservative-free artificial tears and nighttime ophthalmic lubricating ointment, along with punctal occlusion may help restore the ocular surface. Autologous serum tears have shown great potential by increasing corneal sensitivity, providing neurotrophic factors and accelerating epithelial healing in neurotrophic keratopathy. Use of topical steroids is controversial because, although they decrease inflammation of the ocular surface, they can inhibit stromal healing and increase the risk of a corneal melt and perforation which may result in reactivation of the viral keratitis. Commercially available cyclosporine A formulations act to decrease inflammation of the ocular surface and are not associated with corneal melts, but are not as potent as most steroid formulations. It must be remembered that steroids and cyclosporine A can cause an HSV reactivation. For more advanced disease, an amniotic membrane graft may help to heal the ocular surface, which is important since an intact ocular surface is much more resistant to tissue breakdown. Additional advanced therapy may require the use of corneal or scleral therapeutic contact lenses or partial tarsorrhaphy. We have had great success using scleral contact lenses or specialty large contact lenses, such as

Figure 12-4. Chemical injury of the eye. The eye has a complete epithelial defect, an avascular appearance to the limbus, which implies corneal stem cell damage, and inflammation and chemosis of the bulbar conjunctiva, which may signal damage of the accessory lacrimal glands.

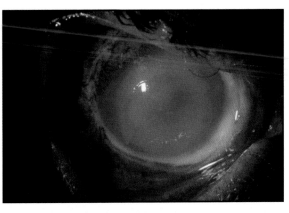

the Prosthetic Replacement of the Ocular Surface Ecosystem (PROSE) treatment, in cases of severe neurotrophic keratopathy. These hard contact lenses can improve vision by correcting the irregular astigmatism induced by the scars of previous viral infections and reducing evaporation from the ocular surface.

CHEMICAL INJURY—RELATED DRY EYE

Chemical injury of the eye may produce extensive permanent damage to the ocular surface. Alkali agents typically penetrate deeper than acids, but the severity of an injury is determined by the surface area of contact and the degree of tissue penetration and damage (Figure 12-4). Recovery of an intact and normal ocular surface is crucial to favorable outcomes following ocular chemical injuries.

Treatment of a chemical injury related to dry eye should promote re-epithelialization and promote repair of the ocular surface. After the emergent condition is stabilized (eg, copious irrigation, removal of particulate chemical matter, debridement of necrotic tissue, topical corticosteroids), the ocular surface may become dry due to an irregular epithelial surface, LCSD, or damage to meibomian glands, goblet cells, and lacrimal glands. After the acute treatment of the injury, frequent preservative-free tears and ointment should be initiated. Moisture chambers or serum tears maybe necessary in severe cases.[27-29] Amniotic membrane transplantation (AMT) can be used in both the acute and chronic setting of chemical injuries to reconstruct the ocular surface, reduce inflammation, and reduce fibrosis. AMT has been shown in some small case studies to reduce the incidence of LCSD after chemical injury, and it may also reduce perilimbal inflammation and corneal neovascularization. Antioxidant vitamins (such as oral and topical ascorbate and citrate), oral doxycycline, and omega-3 fatty acids have also been used during the recovery phase to reduce risk of ulceration. Temporary or permanent tarsorrhaphy may also benefit the ocular surface in refractory cases by reducing evaporation from the ocular surface. Like the tarsorraphy, large scleral contact lenses can be beneficial in certain cases but symblepharon formation may prevent their use. Finally, if the ocular surface is not salvageable and prohibits successful keratoplasty, then a keratoprosthesis, such as the K-Pro type 1 or type 2, is an option for visual rehabilitation. However, they are associated with certain risks and potential complications, so the risks vs benefits must be weighed.

SUMMARY

Any dry eye treatment must address the underlying pathology. As evidenced by the discussion above, there is no single treatment for all disorders. A thorough understanding of the therapeutic options is essential in order to create the best treatment plan.

REFERENCES

1. Whaley K, Buchanan WW. *Clinical Immunology.* Vol 1. Philadelphia, PA: WB Sanders; 1981.
2. Lucca JA, Kung JS, Farris RL. Keratoconjunctivitis sicca in HIV-1 infected female patients. In: Sullivan DA, ed. *Lacrimal Gland, Tear Film and Dry Eye Syndromes.* New York, NY: Plenum; 1994.
3. Parekh M, Poli B, Ferrari S, Teofili C, Ponzin D. *Aniridia: Recent Developments in Scientific and Clinical Research.* Cham, Switzerland: Springer; 2015.
4. Shiple D, Finklea B, Lauderdale JD, Netland PA. Keratopathy, cataract, and dry eye in a survey of aniridia subjects. *Clin Ophthalmol.* 2010;9:291-295.
5. Janstaneiah S, Al-Rajhi AA. Association of aniridia and dry eyes. *Ophthalmology.* 2005;112:1535-1540.
6. Eden U, Fagerholm P, Danyali R, Lagali N. Pathologic epithelial and anterior corneal nerve morphology in early-stage congenital aniridia keratopathy. *Ophthalmology.* 2010;119:1803-1810.
7. Lopez-Garcia, JS, Rivas L, Garcia-Lozano I, Marube J. Autologous serum eyedrops in the treatment of aniridic keratopathy. *Ophthalmology.* 2008;115:262-267.
8. Tan DTH, Ficker LA, Buckley RJ. Limbal transplantation. *Ophthalmology.* 1996;103:29-36.
9. Selter JH, Gire AI, Sikder S. The relationship between Graves' ophthalmopathy and dry eye syndrome. *Clin Ophthalmol.* 2015;9:57-62.
10. McAlinder C. An overview of thyroid eye disease. *Eye and Vision.* 2014;1:9.
11. Bahn RS. Graves' ophthalmopathy. *N Engl J Med.* 2010;362(8):726-738.
12. Kan E, Kilickan E, Ecemis G, et al. Presence of dry eye in patients with Hashimoto's thyroiditis. *J Ophthalmol.* 2014;2014:754923.
13. Eckstein AK, Finkenrath A, Heiligenhaus A. Dry eye syndrome in thyroid-associated ophthalmopathy: lacrimal expression of TSH receptors suggests involvements of TSH-specific autoantibodies. *Acta Ophthalmol.* 2004;82(3):291-297.
14. Cher I. Superior limbic keratoconjunctivitis: multifactorial mechanical pathogenesis. *Clin Exp Ophthalmol.* 2000;28:181-184.
15. Gris O, Plazas A, Lerma E, et al. Conjunctival resection with and without amniotic membrane graft for the treatment of superior limbic keratoconjunctivitis. *Cornea.* 2010;29(9):1025-1030.
16. Chun YS, Kim JC. Treatment of superior limbic keratoconjunctivitis with a large-diameter contact lens and botulium toxin A. *Cornea.* 2009;28(7):752-758.
17. Singh K, Axelrod S, Bielory L. The epidemiology of ocular and nasal allergy in the United States. *J Allergy Clin Immunol.* 2010;126(4):778-783.e6.
18. Vehof J, Smitt-Kamminga NS, Nibourg SA, Hammond CJ. Predictors of discordance between symptoms and signs in dry eye disease. *Ophthalmology.* 2017;124(3):280-286.
19. Ousler GW, Wilcox KA, Gupta G, Abelson MB. An evaluation of the ocular drying effects of 2 systemic antihistamines: loratadine and cetirizine hydrochloride. *Ann Allergy Asthma Immunol.* 2004;93:460-464.
20. Bonini S, Rama P, Olzi D, Lambiase A. Neurotrophic keratitis. *Eye.* 2003;17:989-995.
21. Hill GM, Ku ES, Dwarakanathan S. Herpes simplex keratitis. *Disease-a-Month.* 2014;60:239-246.

22. Kaufman SC. Anterior segment complications of herpes zoster virus ophthalmicus. *Ophthalmology.* 2008;115:S24-S32.

23. Liesegang TJ. Herpes zoster ophthalmicus. *Ophthalmology.* 2008;115:S3-S12.

24. Matsumoto Y, Dogru M, Goto E, et al. Autologous serum application in the treatment of neurotrophic keratopathy. *Ophthalmology.* 2004;111:1115-1120.

25. Rowe A, Leger AS, Jeon S, Dhaliwal DK, Knickelbein JE, Hendricks RL. Herpes keratitis. *Prog Retin Eye Res.* 2013;32C:88-101.

26. Sacchetti M, Lambiase A. Diagnosis and management of neurotrophic keratitis. *Clin Ophthalmol.* 2014;8:517-579.

27. Fish R, Davidson RS. Management of ocular thermal and chemical injuries, including amniotic membrane therapy. *Curr Opin Ophthalmol.* 2010;21:317-321.

28. Sharma N, Kaur M, Agarwal T, Sangwan VS, Vajpayee RB. Treatment of acute ocular chemical burns. *Surv Ophthalmol.* 2018;63(2):214-235.

29. Wagoner MD. Chemical injuries of the eye: current concepts in pathophysiology and therapy. *Surv Ophthalmol.* 1997;41:275-313.

CHAPTER 13

The Dermatologic Patient
Rosacea, Stevens-Johnson Syndrome, and Isotretinoin

Patricia B. Sierra, MD

KEY POINTS

- Ocular manifestations, most commonly blepharitis, occur in about 50% of patients with rosacea at some point in the course of their disease. Corneal involvement in the form of a superficial punctate keratopathy with a marginal vascular infiltrate occur in 5% to 30% of patients.
- Once-daily, low-dose doxycycline (40 mg) has been gaining popularity in the treatment of ocular rosacea.
- Stevens-Johnson syndrome (SJS) and toxic epidermal necrolysis (TEN) are severe immunologic dermatobullous conditions with high mortality. Drugs such as sulfonamide antibiotics and infections are the most frequent identifiable precipitating factors.
- Bilateral conjunctivitis occurs in 15% to 75% of patients with SJS. Severe cicatrization of the conjunctiva with symblepharon formation, entropion, trichiasis, and tear film instability may occur. Lacrimal duct scarring and conjunctival goblet cell destruction may lead to a severe dry eye state.
- Early ophthalmic evaluation and aggressive treatment in SJS is essential to decelerate disease progression and reduce the likelihood of long-term complications.
- Amniotic membrane transplantation (AMT) is becoming the gold standard in the management of acute SJS/TEN.
- Oral isotretinoin is a Vitamin A analogue in the treatment of acne vulgaris. For patients treated with isotretinoin, 30% complain of dry eye related to meibomian gland atrophy. Variable presentation of corneal deposits can also occur (fine, rounded, subepithelial white to gray lesions).

Mah FS, Rhee MK, eds.
Dry Eye Disease: A Practical Guide (pp 133-142).
© 2019 Taylor & Francis Group.

Figure 13-1. Roseatic facies with evident ocular involvement. Note the characteristic erythema, papules, pustules, and telangiectasia of the face and eyelid and conjunctival involvement.

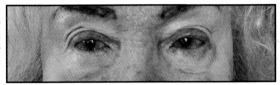

Figure 13-2. Eyelid erythema and thickening associated with rosacea.

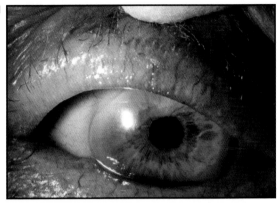

ROSACEA

Rosacea is a common, chronic, inflammatory dermatosis that predominantly involves the flush areas of the face (forehead, nose and cheeks). It may affect up to 10% of the population and occurs mostly in middle-aged and older individuals.[1] The facial skin lesions are characterized by erythema, papules, pustules, and telangiectasia (Figure 13-1).

Ocular manifestations occur in about 50% of patients with rosacea at some point in the course of their disease.[2] Skin findings usually precede the eye findings, but on occasion, the eye may be affected first. The eyelids, conjunctiva, cornea, and episclera may be involved. Blepharitis, meibomian gland dysfunction,[3] conjunctival hyperemia, and dry eye are the most common associated findings.[4,5] The eyelid margins are hyperemic, thickened, and telangiectatic (Figure 13-2). The meibomian glands secrete excess sebum, and the orifices may be inspissated and inflamed. The conjunctiva can become injected with vascular dilation and edema.

Corneal involvement can be seen in approximately 5% to 30% of cutaneous rosacea patients.[6] A superficial punctate keratopathy is common and a marginal vascular infiltration can occur in the peripheral cornea. As the keratitis progresses, subepithelial infiltrates can form at the leading edge of "spade-shaped" pannus, which are usually inferior and can be associated with scarring and stromal thinning (Figure 13-3).

The etiology of rosacea is unknown. Vasomotor lability is easily induced and appears to be aggravated by coffee, tea, alcohol, spicy foods, endocrine abnormalities, menopause, and anxiety. Studies show elevated matrix metalloproteinase-9 in the conjunctival epithelium.[7]

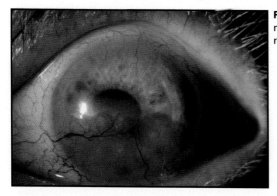

Figure 13-3. Severe corneal marginal neovascularization secondary to chronic rosacea.

The treatment of rosacea begins with avoidance of food, beverages, and environments that exacerbate flushing. Both cutaneous and ocular rosacea respond well to oral tetracycline, doxycycline, or azithromycin.[8]

Treatment of ocular rosacea has historically been 50 to 100 mg of doxycycline twice daily.[9,10] However, the use of once-daily, low-dose doxycycline (40 mg) has been gaining popularity to prevent common side effects.[11] Additional measures such as eyelid hygiene, heat application, and massage can help control the blepharitis. Preservative-free artificial tears and antibiotic and steroid application can improve conjunctivitis and keratitis. If corneal ulceration is present, microbial involvement must be ruled out. Corticosteroids must be used judiciously, as some patients may be susceptible to corneal melt and perforation.

Topical metronidazole cream and gel are beneficial to help maintain remission for cutaneous rosacea.

STEVENS-JOHNSON SYNDROME

The spectrum of diseases defined by Stevens-Johnson syndrome (SJS), the more severe toxic epidermal necrolysis (TEN), and their intermediate SJS/TEN overlap are severe immunologic dermatobullous conditions with high mortality and significant long-term morbidity. SJS/TEN is characterized by widespread keratinocyte death and epidermal necrosis resulting in splitting of subepidermal layers with attendant tissue loss at skin and mucosal surfaces.[12]

SJS was first described by 2 American physicians, Stevens and Johnson, who reported 2 classic cases in children and named the disease eruptive fever with stomatitis and ophthalmia in 1922.[13] The estimated annual incidence (cases/million; population/ year) of SJS/TEN ranges from 0.4 to 7 cases per million population, making it a rare disease.[14,15]

PRESENTATION

Drugs and infections are the most frequent identifiable precipitating factors. Common medications associated with SJS/TEN include sulfonamide antibiotics (trimethoprim/sulfamethoxazole), aromatic anticonvulsants (eg, phenytoin, phenobarbital, and carbamazepine), beta-lactam antibiotics, nevirapine, abacavir, nonsteroidal antiinflammatory medications, allopurinol, lamotrigine, tetracyclines, quinolones, and others.[16]

Initial symptoms in SJS can include high fever, muscular pain, nausea, vomiting, diarrhea, migratory arthralgias, and pharyngitis. Within days, the typical dermatologic and mucosal lesions begin to break out. Two or more mucosal surfaces are involved, including the conjunctiva, oral cavity, upper airway or esophagus, gastrointestinal tract, or anogenital mucosa. Skin involvement is typically less than 20% of the total body surface area in SJS. Depending on the extent of the bullae, associated risks include significant blood and insensible fluid loss, as well as a high risk of bacterial superinfection and sepsis. The disorder is usually self-limited, with a typical total duration of 4 to 6 weeks.

OCULAR FINDINGS

The ocular complications are generally acknowledged as the most debilitating residual effects of SJS/TEN. Ocular involvement in the acute phase of SJS/TEN occurs due to rapid-onset keratinocyte apoptosis and secondary effects of inflammation and loss of ocular surface epithelium. Acute ocular involvement is reported to occur in 50% to 88% of SJS/TEN cases. Early involvement is highly variable and can range from self-limited conjunctival hyperemia to near total sloughing of the entire ocular surface epithelium, including the tarsal conjunctiva and eyelid margin.[17]

Initially, a nonspecific conjunctivitis usually occurs at the same time as lesions on the skin and other mucous membranes. The conjunctivitis may, however, precede the skin eruption. The bilateral conjunctivitis may be catarrhal or pseudomembranous and occurs in 15% to 75% of patients with SJS.[18] Secondary purulent bacterial conjunctivitis can complicate the initial ocular involvement. In some patients, a severe anterior uveitis may occur. Uncommonly, corneal ulceration can occur during the acute stage of the disease.

The initial eye findings usually resolve in 2 to 4 weeks but, unfortunately, the inflammatory reaction can result in severe cicatrization of the conjunctiva with symblepharon formation, entropion, trichiasis, and instability of the tear film.[19] Subsequent breakdown of the ocular surface induces corneal scarring, neovascularization, and, in severe cases, keratinization (Figure 13-4). Keratin often accumulates, not only on the corneal surface, but also along the posterior eyelid margin, further abrading the ocular surface and potentially leading to persistent epithelial defects. Cicatrization of the lacrimal ducts in association with destruction of the conjunctival goblet cells may lead to a severe dry eye state. The degree of corneal scarring correlates with the severity of eyelid margin and tarsal pathology.[20]

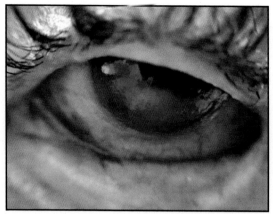

Figure 13-4. Corneal and conjunctival keratinization following SJS. (Reprinted with permission from Jennifer Li, MD.)

MANAGEMENT

Ophthalmologists should play a central role in the early evaluation and treatment of patients with SJS/TEN. Every patient thought to have acute SJS/TEN should have prompt ophthalmic evaluation and aggressive ophthalmic treatment which is essential to decelerate disease progression and reduce the likelihood of long-term complications.

The entire ocular surface should be carefully examined. The examination should always include fluorescein staining to detect and document membranes and denuded epithelium. Any patient with eyelid margin involvement, conjunctival pseudomembranes, apposing bulbar and tarsal conjunctival defects, or corneal epithelial defects should be evaluated daily during the acute stage.

Preservative free artificial tears, ocular antibiotics, and topical anti-inflammatory medications should be used frequently in the acute stage of SJS/TEN. Corticosteroid ointment should be applied to the eyelid margins, and topical corticosteroid solution or suspension to the eye surface on a frequent basis (at least 3 to 6 times per day), except in cases of concurrent microbial keratitis.

Cryopreserved amniotic membrane transplantation (AMT) is becoming the gold standard in the management of acute SJS/TEN. The amniotic membrane (AM) serves as a biological bandage by suppressing inflammation, promoting epithelialization, and thereby preventing sight-threatening sequelae. To obtain the best possible outcomes with AMT, it is important to completely cover the entire ocular surface and eyelid margins with amnion and as early in the clinical course as possible. Ideally, AMT should be performed within 5 days of onset of SJS/TEN. AM typically dissolves over a period of 1 to 2 weeks; thus, more than 1 application may be necessary during the acute phase of the disease.[21]

A simple grading system adapted from Sotozono and coworkers and suggested management is shown in Table 13-1. Epithelial sloughing of the ocular surface and/or eyelid margin, or pseudomembrane formation, are indications for AMT, in addition to aggressive lubrication, topical antibiotic, and corticosteroid therapy.[22] Ma et al described a

TABLE 13-1

GRADING SCORES FOR ACUTE OCULAR SEVERITY OF STEVENS-JOHNSON SYNDROME AND TOXIC EPIDERMAL NECROLYSIS

ACUTE OCULAR MANIFESTATIONS	GRADE	MANAGEMENT
No ocular involvement	0 (none)	AT 4 times a day
Conjunctival hyperemia	1 (mild)	AT every hour Topical antibiotic Topical steroids
Either ocular surface epithelial defect or pseudomembrane formation	2 (severe)	Above therapies plus AMT
Both ocular surface epithelial defect and pseudomembrane formation	3 (very severe)	Above therapies plus AMT

Abbreviations: AT = artificial tears; AMT = amniotic membrane transplantation.

Adapted from Kohanim S, Palioura S, Saeed H, et al. Acute and chronic opththalmic involvement in Stevens-Johnson syndrome/toxic epidermal necrolysis - a comprehensive review and guide to therapy. II. Ophthalmic disease. *Ocul Surf.* 2016;14:168-188 and Sotozono C, Ueta M, Nakatani E, et al. Predictive factors associated with acute ocular involvement in Stevens-Johnson syndrome and toxic epidermal necrolysis. *Am J Ophthalmol.* 2015;160:228-237.

technique for placement of single, large sheet of AM (5 x 10 cm) and a custom-made forniceal ring for AMT in ocular SJS (Figure 13-5).[23]

Following the initial acute stage, recognizing the complications of trichiasis, epithelial surface disease, keratinization of the eyelid margins and secondary infection can improve the outcome.

Eyelid malpositions, lagophthalmus, misdirected eyelashes, and keratinization of eyelid margins should be addressed by surgical intervention and/ or mucous membrane grafting.

Ocular surface disease and persistent epithelial defects should be treated aggressively with non-preserved artificial tears and ointment, discontinuance of toxic topical medications, punctal occlusion, autologous serum, AM, and/or scleral contact lens placement.[24]

If the ocular surface is severely damage with limbal stem cell deficiency and corneal neovascularization, management becomes particularly challenging due to frequent failure of keratolimbal allografts in SJS/TEN patients.[25] Keratoprosthesis implantation can provide hope for the most severely affected but should be considered only as a last resort due to decreased retention and increased complications in these patients.[26]

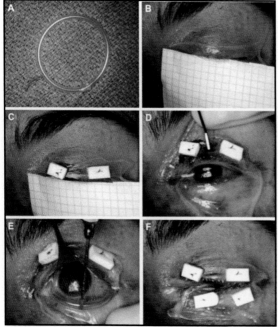

Figure 13-5. AM transplantation utilizing a single 5 x 10 cm sheet. (A) Creation of symblepharon ring with intravenous tubing. (B) Placement of AM over upper eyelid. (C) Anchoring of AM using 6-0 polypropylene mattress sutures and bolsters. (D) Unfolding of AM over the ocular surface. (E) Placement of the custom-made symblepharon ring in the fornices. The ring is already pushed into the upper fornix and is being gently deposited into the lower fornix. (F) Anchoring of AM to lower eyelid. (Reprinted with permission from Ma KN, Thanos A, Chodosh J, Shah AS, Mantagos IS. A novel technique for amniotic membrane transplantation in patients with acute stevens-johnson syndrome. *Ocul Surf.* 2016;14(1):31-36.)

ORAL ISOTRETINOIN

Isotretinoin (Accutane) is a Vitamin A analogue that has revolutionized the treatment of acne vulgaris over the past 25 years as a result of its high efficacy and the prolonged remission achieved with this therapy.[27] In the skin, it is known to cause atrophic changes in the sebaceous gland acini with a marked decrease in sebum production.

Ocular findings are among the more frequent side effects in patients taking isotretinoin. The most common adverse ocular effect is blepharoconjunctivitis, with dry eyes being a complaint of 30% of patients treated.[28] Other side effects include blurred vision, photophobia, contact lens intolerance, corneal infiltrates, and opacities which appear to be dose dependent.[29,30]

Corneal deposits can have variable presentations and can be fine, rounded, sub-epithelial, or contain white to gray lesions of various sizes in the central or peripheral cornea. The lesions usually do not stain with fluorescein but can have some epithelial irregularity over the involved area. Visual loss can occur if the visual axis is involved. These opacities are more common in patients who wear contact lenses and usually resolve with discontinuation of therapy, but there are reports of long lasting, persistent corneal abnormalities (Figure 13-6).

Various studies have attempted to explain the etiology of the ocular surface side effects and a lipid deficiency has been well-established. Mathers et al[31] demonstrated that increased tear osmolarity with the use of oral isotretinoin is a result of meibomian gland atrophy and that the consequent lipo-deficiency leads to changes in the tear

Figure 13-6. Corneal opacities and nodules in a patient with a history of isotretinoin and contact lens use.

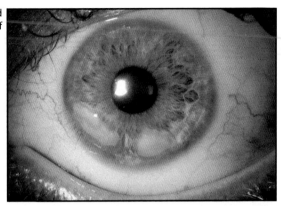

Figure 13-7. Meibomian gland dropout associated with isotretinoin use.

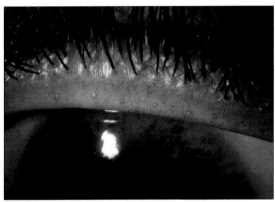

film evaporation rate (Figure 13-7). During their study, meibomian glands appeared significantly less dense and atrophic by meibography. Such atrophy leads to a decrease in lipid secretion and destabilization of the tear film. These investigators also found no significant changes in Schirmer test in these same patients; hence, an absence of any associated aqueous deficiency. Isotretinoin was also found to decrease goblet cell density inducing a mucin deficiency in another study.[32]

Other more serious ocular side effects reported include papilledema or pseudotumor cerebri, optic neuritis, myopia, decreased dark adaptation, and intraocular inflammation (uveitis, scleritis, retinitis, iritis). Development of these conditions demands discontinuation of the drug. Patients with dry eyes should be monitored closely and in those with corneal opacities, prudence indicates reduction of the dosage or discontinuation of isotretinoin.[28]

REFERENCES

1. Wilkin JK. Rosacea. Pathophysiology and treatment. *Arch Dermatol.* 1994;130:359.
2. Starr PAJ, McDonald A. Oculocutaneous aspects of rosacea. *Proc R Soc Med.* 1969;62:9.
3. Palamar M, Degirmenci C, Ertam I, Yagci A. Evaluation of dry eye and meibomian gland dysfunction with meibography in patients with rosacea. *Cornea.* 2015;34:497-499.
4. Wise G. Ocular rosacea. *Am J Ophthalmol.* 1943;26:591-609.
5. Ghanem VC, Mehra N, Wong S, et al. The prevalence of ocular signs in acne rosacea: comparing patients from ophthalmology and dermatology clinics. *Cornea.* 2003;22:230-233.
6. Thygeson P. Dermatoses with ocular manifestations. In: Sorsby A, ed. *Systemic ophthalmology.* 2nd ed. London: Butterworths; 1958.
7. Maatta M, et al.Tear fluid levels of MMP-8 are elevated in ocular rosacea-treatment effect of oral doxycycline. *Graefe's Arch Clin Exp Ophthalmol.* 2006;244:957.
8. Sneddon IB. A clinical trial of tetracycline in rosacea. *Br J Dermatol.* 1966;78:649.
9. Tanzi EL, Weinberg JM. The ocular manifestations of rosacea. *Cutis.* 2001;68:112-114.
10. Jenkins MS, et al. Ocular rosacea. *Am J Ophthalmol.* 1979;88:1618.
11. Sobolewska B, Doycheva D, Deuter C, et al. Treatment of Ocular Rosacea with Once-Daily Low-Dose Doxycycline. *Cornea.* 2014;33:257-260.
12. Letko, E, Papaliodis, DN, Papaliodis, GN et al. Stevens-Johnson syndrome and toxic epidermal necrolysis: a review of the literature. *Ann Allergy Asthma Immunol.* 2005;94:419-436.
13. Stevens AM, Johnson FC. A new eruptive fever associated with stomatitis and ophthalmia. *Am J Dis Child.* 1922;24:526-533.
14. Roujeau JC, et al. Toxic epidermal necrolysis (Lyell syndrome). Incidence and drug etiology in France, 1981-1985. *Arch Dermatol.* 1990;126:37-42.
15. Griggs, R.C., Batshaw, M., Dunkle, M. et al. Clinical research for rare disease: opportunities, challenges, and solutions. *Mol Genet Metab.* 2009;96:20-26.
16. Letko, E., Papaliodis, D.N., Papaliodis, GN et al. Stevens-Johnson syndrome and toxic epidermal necrolysis: a review of the literature. *Ann Allergy Asthma Immunol.* 2005;94:419-436.
17. Power, WJ, Ghoraishi, M, Merayo-Lloves, J et al. Analysis of the acute ophthalmic manifestations of the erythema multiforme/Stevens-Johnson syndrome/toxic epidermal necrolysis disease spectrum. *Ophthalmology.* 1995;102:1669-1676.
18. Howard GM. The Stevens-Johnson syndrome. Ocular prognosis and treatment. *Am J Ophthalmol.* 1963;55:893-900.
19. Arstikaitis, MJ. Ocular aftermath of Stevens-Johnson syndrome. *Arch Ophthalmol.* 1973;90:376-379.
20. Di Pascuale, MA, Espana, EM, Liu, DT et al. Correlation of corneal complications with eyelid cicatricial pathologies in patients with Stevens-Johnson syndrome and toxic epidermal necrolysis syndrome. *Ophthalmology.* 2005;112:904-912.
21. Kohanim S, Palioura S, Saeed H, et al. Acute and chronic opththalmic involvement in Stevens-Johnson syndrome/toxic epidermal necrolysis - a comprehensive review and guide to therapy. II. Ophthalmic disease. *Ocul Surf.* 2016;14:168-188
22. Sotozono, C, Ueta, M, Nakatani, E, et al. Predictive factors associated with acute ocular involvement in Stevens-Johnson syndrome and toxic epidermal necrolysis. *Am J Ophthalmol.* 2015;160:228-237.
23. Ma KN, Thanos A, Chodosh J, et al. A Novel Technique for Amniotic Membrane Transplantation in Patients with Acute Stevens-Johnson Syndrome. *Ocul Surf.* 2016;14:31-36.
24. Papakostas, TD, Le, HG, Chodosh, J, Jacobs, DS. Prosthetic replacement of the ocular surface ecosystem as treatment for ocular surface disease in patients with a history of Stevens-Johnson syndrome/toxic epidermal necrolysis. *Ophthalmology.* 2015;122:248-253.
25. Solomon, A, Ellies, P, Anderson, DF, et al. Long-term outcome of keratolimbal allograft with or without penetrating keratoplasty for total limbal stem cell deficiency. *Ophthalmology.* 2002;109:1159-1166.
26. Robert, MC and Dohlman, CH. A review of corneal melting after Boston Keratoprosthesis. *Semin Ophthalmol.* 2014;29:349-357.
27. Zouboulis CC. Isotretinoin revisited: pluripotent effects on human sebaceous gland cells. *J Invest Dermatol.* 2006;126(10):2154-2156.

28. Fraunfelder FT, LaBraico JM, Meyer SM. Adverse ocular reactions possibly associated with isotretinoin. *Am J Ophthalmol*. 1985;100:534-537.

29. Fraunfelder FT, LaBraico JM, Meyer SM. Adverse ocular reactions possibly associated with isotretinoin. *Am J Ophthalmol*. 1985;100:534-537.

30. Weiss J, Degnan M. Leupold R, Lumpkin LR. Bilateral corneal opacities: occurrence in a patient treated with oral isotretinoin. *Arch Dermatol*. 1981;117:182-183.

31. Mathers WD, Shields WJ, Sachdev MS, et al. Meibomian gland morphology and tear osmolarity: changes with accutane therapy. *Cornea*. 1991;10:286-290.

32. De Queiroga IBW, Antonio Vieira L, Barros JN, et al. Conjunctival Impression Cytology Changes Induced by Oral Isotretinoin. *Cornea*. 2009;28:1009-1013.

CHAPTER 14

The Surgical Patient

Kourtney Houser, MD and Stephen C. Pflugfelder, MD

KEY POINTS

- Attention to and management of dry eye is critical in the surgical patient, especially in multifocal intraocular lens (IOL) patients.
- A smooth and stable tear layer is essential for maintaining high quality vision between blinks, as the tear/corneal epithelial complex accounts for about 65% of the eye's optical power.
- Dry eye can lead to errors in IOL selection and resultant refractive surprises since tear film instability impedes accurate keratometry, topography, and biometry.

The tear/corneal epithelial complex is the major light refracting surface of the eye, accounting for approximately 65% of the eye's optical power. A smooth and stable tear layer is essential for maintaining high-quality vision between blinks.[1] Significant ocular surface disease has the potential to worsen outcomes in vision correcting surgery if not managed appropriately preoperatively and postoperatively. New or worsened dry eye disease following refractive procedures and cataract surgery are common and can lead to patient dissatisfaction.[2-4]

Mah FS, Rhee MK, eds.
Dry Eye Disease: A Practical Guide (pp 143-154).
© 2019 Taylor & Francis Group.

Attention to and management of dry eye perioperatively in cataract patients is important, as dry eye is common in this age group. Dry eye not only affects visual quality following cataract surgery due to the ocular surface itself, but can also lead to errors in intraocular lens (IOL) selection and resultant refractive surprises. Tear film instability adversely affects keratometric measurements, which rely on a good quality corneal surface for accurate readings. Tear instability and hyperosmolarity from dry eye is associated with poor repeatability of keratometry readings that can result in inaccurate IOL power calculations.[5] Residual ametropia, often caused or worsened by dry eye, is especially detrimental to patient satisfaction following multifocal IOL implantation.[6-8] Appropriate treatment of the ocular surface prior to preoperative topography and biometry is critical to ensure consistent axis and magnitude of keratometry readings that are necessary for proper lens selection. If a toric multifocal lens is not selected, but significant astigmatism is present, astigmatism management at the time of IOL implantation, or subsequently, may be necessary to maximize visual acuity and patient satisfaction.[9]

Results of corneal refractive surgery can also be adversely affected by dry eye. Ocular dryness commonly occurs after LASIK, and most studies suggest photorefractive keratectomy (PRK) carries a lower risk of developing dry eye signs and symptoms in the early postop period than LASIK.[10-12] The impact of LASIK on the ocular surface is likely due to a combination of decreased corneal innervation, disruption to the lacrimal functional unit, decreased tear secretion, and decreased goblet cell density.[7,13,14] The resulting dry eye adversely affects patient satisfaction and visual function. Additionally, significantly more regression following myopic LASIK has been reported in patients with chronic dry eye.[15] Furthermore, aggressive treatment of dry eye is necessary to maximize patient satisfaction and visual function.

DRY EYE AND MULTIFOCAL INTRAOCULAR LENS SELECTION

Ocular surface evaluation and management is of particular importance in patients considering cataract surgery with multifocal IOL implantation. While dry eye does not preclude patients from multifocal implantation, preoperative management of symptoms and signs and thorough counseling is critical for successful outcomes. Ocular surface health should be maximized prior to taking preoperative keratotomy measurements, and patients must be aware that long-term treatment regimens may be required to optimize visual function when this type of lens is implanted. Patient selection is very important and tear dysfunction should be managed on a case-by-case basis.[16] Diagnosis and treatment of tear dysfunction should be initiated preoperatively, especially since uncomplicated phacoemulsification and postoperative topical therapies may temporarily worsen signs and symptoms of dry eye and increase the risk of complications.[16,17]

Patient dissatisfaction following implantation of multifocal IOLs typically results from perceptions of glare, halos, decreased night vision, reduced contrast sensitivity, and photic phenomena.[18-21] Dry eye is an important source of these visual complaints that should not be overlooked. In a retrospective review of 44 consecutive patients presenting with visual complaints following multifocal implantation, 15% of those complaining of blurry vision and 5% experiencing photic phenomenon had dry eye as the etiology of their symptoms.[8]

DIAGNOSTIC APPROACH TO THE SURGICAL CANDIDATE

A 45-year-old female with a history of hyperopia (+2.00 in both eyes), 15 years of soft contact lens use, recent contact lens intolerance, and dry eyes presents for refractive surgery evaluation. She uses artificial tears occasionally, which provide temporary improvement in her dry eye symptoms. Her past medical history is significant for adolescent nodular acne treated for 1 year with isotretinoin approximately 20 years ago.

In a patient like this, thorough preoperative screening is essential to determine if the patient is a good candidate for surgery and for maximizing patient safety and satisfaction.[22] Many patients who seek refractive surgery do so because of intolerance to contact lenses, which often occurs due to aging and ocular surface changes, such as goblet cell loss and meibomian gland disease that can develop from chronic contact lens use or over wear. Preexisting dry eye is a strong predictor of chronic and more severe dry eye after surgery, as well as slowed recovery of corneal sensitivity that increases the risk of developing neurotrophic epitheliopathy.[4,23,24] Many patients with preexisting dry eye symptoms may have an improvement in symptoms several months after LASIK; however, a small percentage of previously asymptomatic patients may develop moderate or severe dry eye symptoms following the procedure.[25] Therefore, it is important that all patients are counseled about dry eye, even if they are asymptomatic preoperatively.

History of prior diseases that could contribute to the development of neurotrophic keratopathy should be elicited, including history of herpes zoster ophthalmicus or herpes simplex virus keratitis. History should also include inquiry about autoimmune diseases, such as Sjögren syndrome and rheumatoid arthritis. These patients, even if asymptomatic and with a normal exam, could progress to refractory dry eye with aging and this could be accelerated by LASIK.[26]

History of medications, especially isotretinoin use, should be obtained. Isotretinoin has many known ocular side effects, including meibomian gland atrophy and dysfunction, tear instability, ocular discomfort, blepharoconjunctivitis, and photophobia.[27,28] The potential impacts of this medication on the ocular surface and on dry eye symptoms should be discussed with patients. Additionally, medications with anticholinergic side effects, such as antihistamines and antidepressants, should be identified.

Accurate manifest and cycloplegic refractions, which require a stable tear film, must be obtained preoperatively to ensure proper treatment selection. Compared to myopic corrections, more peripheral ablation is required for treating hyperopia, and this increases the risk of corneal hypoesthesia and dry eye.[29] Higher refractive corrections with deeper ablation depths also increase the risk of developing dry eye.[3,30,31]

A systematic approach, such as the one shown in Figure 14-1, should be taken to diagnose tear dysfunction preoperatively. Slit-lamp examination can yield valuable

Figure 14-1. Suggested diagnostic approach for patient considering keratorefractive or cataract surgery. MGD = meibomian gland dysfunction.

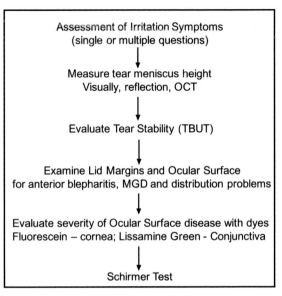

Assessment of Irritation Symptoms
(single or multiple questions)

↓

Measure tear meniscus height
Visually, reflection, OCT

↓

Evaluate Tear Stability (TBUT)

↓

Examine Lid Margins and Ocular Surface
for anterior blepharitis, MGD and distribution problems

↓

Evaluate severity of Ocular Surface disease with dyes
Fluorescein – cornea; Lissamine Green - Conjunctiva

↓

Schirmer Test

information regarding the etiology and severity of dry eye. Eyelids should be examined for eyelash crusting and for signs of meibomian gland disease that include abnormal gland secretions, plugged orifices, increased margin vascularity and irregularity, and tear instability due to lipid deficiency that can result in increased tear evaporation and inflammation of the ocular surface.

Tear film volume and stability should be evaluated and severity of ocular surface disease closely examined with diagnostic dyes. Fluorescein is the best dye to visualize cornea disease, while lissamine green is recommended to detect staining of the conjunctiva. Staining of the cornea and conjunctiva increases with disease severity and can be quantified using grading schemes such as the SICCA Ocular Staining Score.[32] Tear break-up time (TBUT) of less than 10 seconds is indicative of tear film instability, which can persist for months after LASIK.[3,11] Tear volume can be quantified with reflective meniscography or optical coherence tomography (OCT) and tear production by Schirmer testing. Without anesthetic, Schirmer scores 10 mm or less at 5 minutes are considered to be abnormal.[26,33] Quantitative measurement of corneal sensitivity with the Cochet-Bonnet esthesiometer can also be useful in preoperative decision making.

Accurate topography is an essential component of the preoperative evaluation of refractive surgery candidates to assist in the recognition and diagnosis of subclinical and manifest ectasia, as well as other ocular surface abnormalities that may preclude a patient from safe surgery.[34] It is of paramount importance that patients refrain from wearing soft contact lenses for an adequate time period prior to screening and preoperative visits in order to obtain accurate keratometry and ocular surface exams. The time required for the cornea to return to its native contour varies, ranging from 2 to 7 days for daily-wear soft contact lenses, to 1 to 2 weeks for extended-wear soft contact lenses and 6 weeks or longer for rigid contact lenses.[35,36] Irregular astigmatism, asymmetry or pseudokeratoconus can be induced by contact lens wear and/or dry eye and may misguide decision-making and counseling.[37,38] Topography also gives useful information about the quality of the tear film and ocular surface. A Klyce surface regularity index (SRI) 0.80 or more or a surface asymmetry index (SAI) of 0.50 or more have been shown to be sensitive and specific in predicting severity of corneal epithelial disease measured by fluorescein staining.[37]

Anterior segment OCT is a useful and sensitive adjunct test for obtaining corneal thickness maps to screen for ectasia risk in LASIK evaluation.[39] It is useful for measuring the tear meniscus height as a surrogate for tear volume, and tear meniscus height has been shown to correlate with tear break-up time, as well as severity of corneal fluorescein staining.[40,41] A tear meniscus height more than 300 microns has been shown to be sensitive and specific for diagnosing dry eye.[42]

Tear osmolarity has become an objective and widely utilized tool for evaluation of dry eye disease. Meta-analysis has determined that the recommended threshold for diagnosis of dry eye disease to be 316 mOsm/mL (some experts state as low as 308 mOsm/mL) or a variance between eyes of more than 8 mOsm/mL.[43] While tear film osmolarity is not ideal as a single, all-encompassing test for dry eye, nor does it correlate with changes in signs and symptoms in response to therapy, it may be a useful adjunct when analyzed in conjunction with slit-lamp examination and other testing.[44,45]

CLINICAL FINDINGS

Returning to our patient who is interested in hyperopic LASIK, a comprehensive tear and ocular surface examination detected meibomian gland disease with no expressible meibum from the glands, and telangiectatic vessels around the meibomian gland orifices. Fluorescein TBUT was 3 seconds in the right eye and 6 seconds in the left eye. Punctate epithelial erosions were observed in the inferior cornea of both eyes. Mild fluorescein staining (grade 3 of 15) was noted in the inferior cornea bilaterally. There was mild exposure zone conjunctival lissamine green staining. Schirmer 1 test scores were 9 in both eyes. Corneal sensitivity with the Cochet-Bonnet esthesiometer was 4 in each eye. Tear meniscus height measured with anterior segment OCT was 230 microns in the right eye and 240 microns in the left eye. Tear osmolarity was 315 microns in the right eye and 305 microns in the left eye. Corneal topography shows low (< 1 D) regular astigmatism in each eye, with regular mires and SRI of 0.28 in the right eye and 0.2 in the left eye.

Because the patient has evidence of reduced tear volume and unstable tear film causing moderate corneal epithelial disease, treatment is warranted prior to performing refractive surgery. While preoperative dry eye does not reduce the efficacy or safety of the surgical procedure, it is a risk factor for postoperative dry eye signs and symptoms.[46] The reduced corneal sensitivity in this case may be contributing to the aqueous tear deficiency. Meibomian gland disease is likely related to isotretinoin therapy, which results in lipid deficiency and evaporative dry eye.

For this patient, initial treatment should focus on lubricating the ocular surface through the use of artificial tears and punctal plugs. Many multi-dose artificial tears have non-benzalkonium chloride preservatives that are nontoxic, but preservative free options should be considered to minimize toxicity. Punctal plugs could also increase tear volume in this patient and should be considered, as punctal occlusion has been shown to improve irritation symptoms as well as ocular surface disease following LASIK.[47] Dissolvable intracanalicular plugs were inserted in this patient.

TREATMENT CONSIDERATIONS

Our patient returned in 1 month with slight, but inadequate improvement in symptoms and a minimally changed exam. There is an increasing number of treatment options with different mechanisms of action and reported efficacy for treating symptoms and signs of tear dysfunction that are summarized in Table 14-1. These therapies can be considered for patients considering keratorefractive or cataract surgery. Aggressive treatment with one or more therapies can produce impressive results in cornea surface smoothness as demonstrated in the Figure 14-2. This patient had more severe ocular surface disease than our patient who is considering LASIK surgery, but the beneficial effect on cornea smoothness is easily visualized when the pre- and post-treatment topographic exams are compared.

Two months after the addition of topical cyclosporine A, the patient's ocular surface improved and dry eye symptoms resolved. The patient underwent LASIK in both eyes without complication. The patient used steroid and antibiotics drops for 1 week following surgery and continued the cyclosporine A emulsion. At a 3-month postoperative visit, the patient was doing well without dry eye symptoms or other complaints.

OUTCOMES IN TREATED PATIENTS

Many patients with preexisting dry eye that is treated appropriately and aggressively have successful outcomes from cataract or keratorefractive surgeries. Aggressive treatment of dry eye may both improve refractive outcome and decrease the chance of regression and need for enhancement.[15,23] It has been shown that adjunctive cyclosporine A 0.05% drops may have added benefit in both cataract and corneal refractive surgery. In patients with dry eye treated with artificial tears and cyclosporine A drops prior to and following LASIK, after an initial increase at 1 week, Ocular Surface Disease Index scores decrease compared to baseline sooner than those using artificial tears alone, although results have been variable.[48,49] Similarly, cyclosporine A 0.05% may improve visual outcome following multifocal IOL implantation, if used preoperatively and postoperatively.[50] A stepwise approach that may include use of multiple agents should be taken in treating perioperative dry eye, and if treated aggressively, most patients can have a successful outcome.

TABLE 14-1

Evidence-Based Treatment Recommendations for Tear Dysfunction

Symptom/Sign	Artificial Tears[51]	EFA[52-56]	TCN[57-60]	Corticosteroid[61-65]	CsA[66-68]	Lifitegrast 5%[69-72]
Irritation Symptoms	+	+	+	+	+	+
Tear Instability	+	+	+	+	+	
Corneal Epithelial Disease	+		+	+	+	+
Conjunctival Goblet Cells			+	+	+	

Abbreviations: CsA = cyclosporine A; EFA = nutritional supplementation with essential fatty acids; TCN = tetracycline antibiotic (doxycycline, minocycline).

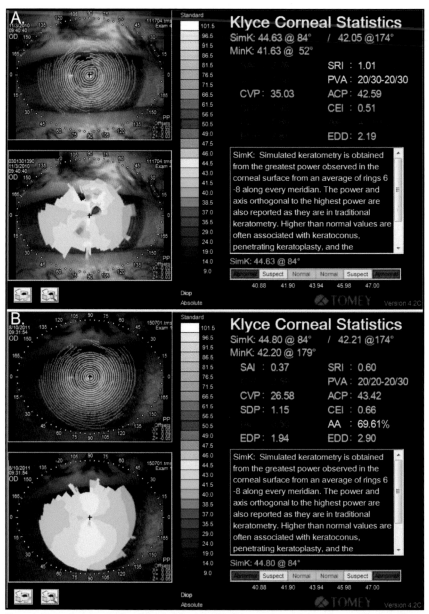

Figure 14-2. Serial cornea topographic examinations in a patient with visually significant nuclear cataract with TBUT of 2 seconds and moderate corneal epithelial disease performed before and after treatment of dry eye. (A) Initial topography examination taken before treatment showing marked irregularity of Placido rings with high SRI and irregular curvature map with asymmetry and skewed astigmatism axis. (B) Exam taken after 9 months of therapy with topical cyclosporine A emulsion, oral doxycycline, and essential fatty acid supplements showing marked improvement in regularity of the reflected rings, SRI and distinct astigmatism axis.

SUMMARY

Clinicians should be vigilant about diagnosing and treating dry eye/tear dysfunction in keratorefractive and cataract surgery candidates, particularly when a toric or multifocal IOL is considered. Tear instability and corneal epithelial disease can influence accuracy of keratometry readings and IOL power calculations and adversely impact visual outcomes and patient satisfaction. There is an increasing number of therapeutic options for improving tear stability and symptoms and signs of dry eye.

REFERENCES

1. Pflugfelder SC. Tear dysfunction and the cornea: LXVIII Edward Jackson Memorial Lecture. *Am J Ophthalmol*. 2011;152(6):900-909.e901.
2. Li XM, Hu L, Hu J, Wang W. Investigation of dry eye disease and analysis of the pathogenic factors in patients after cataract surgery. *Cornea*. 2007;26(9 Suppl 1):S16-20.
3. Battat L, Macri A, Dursun D, Pflugfelder SC. Effects of laser in situ keratomileusis on tear production, clearance, and the ocular surface. *Ophthalmol*. 2001;108(7):1230-1235.
4. Chao C, Golebiowski B, Stapleton F. The role of corneal innervation in LASIK-induced neuropathic dry eye. *Ocul Surf*. 2014;12(1):32-45.
5. Epitropoulos AT, Matossian C, Berdy GJ, Malhotra RP, Potvin R. Effect of tear osmolarity on repeatability of keratometry for cataract surgery planning. *J Cataract Refract Surg*. 2015;41(8):1672-1677.
6. Jabbur NS, Sakatani K, O'Brien TP. Survey of complications and recommendations for management in dissatisfied patients seeking a consultation after refractive surgery. *J Cataract Refract Surg*. 2004;30(9):1867-1874.
7. Lee JB, Ryu CH, Kim J, Kim EK, Kim HB. Comparison of tear secretion and tear film instability after photorefractive keratectomy and laser in situ keratomileusis. *J Cataract Refract Surg*. 2000;26(9):1326-1331.
8. Woodward MA, Randleman JB, Stulting RD. Dissatisfaction after multifocal intraocular lens implantation. *J Cataract Refract Surg*. 2009;35(6):992-997.
9. McNeely RN, Pazo E, Millar Z, et al. Threshold limit of postoperative astigmatism for patient satisfaction after refractive lens exchange and multifocal intraocular lens implantation. *J Cataract Refract Surg*. 2016;42(8):1126-1134.
10. Bower KS, Sia RK, Ryan DS, Mines MJ, Dartt DA. Chronic dry eye in photorefractive keratectomy and laser in situ keratomileusis: Manifestations, incidence, and predictive factors. *J Cataract Refract Surg*. 2015;41(12):2624-2634.
11. Nettune GR, Pflugfelder SC. Post-LASIK tear dysfunction and dysesthesia. *Ocul Surf*. 2010;8(3):135-145.
12. Hovanesian JA, Shah SS, Maloney RK. Symptoms of dry eye and recurrent erosion syndrome after refractive surgery. *J Cataract Refract Surg*. 2001;27(4):577-584.
13. Ryan DS, Bower KS, Sia RK, et al. Goblet cell response after photorefractive keratectomy and laser in situ keratomileusis. *J Cataract Refract Surg*. 2016;42(8):1181-1189.
14. Quinto GG, Camacho W, Behrens A. Postrefractive surgery dry eye. *Curr Opin Ophthalmol*. 2008;19(4):335-341.
15. Albietz JM, Lenton LM, McLennan SG. Chronic dry eye and regression after laser in situ keratomileusis for myopia. *J Cataract Refract Surg*. 2004;30(3):675-684.
16. Kim P, Plugfelder S, Slomovic AR. Top 5 pearls to consider when implanting advanced-technology IOLs in patients with ocular surface disease. *Int Ophthalmol Clin*. 2012;52(2):51-58.
17. Cetinkaya S, Mestan E, Acir NO, Cetinkaya YF, Dadaci Z, Yener HI. The course of dry eye after phacoemulsification surgery. *BMC Ophthalmol*. 2015;15:68.
18. Pepose JS, Qazi MA, Davies J, et al. Visual performance of patients with bilateral vs combination Crystalens, ReZoom, and ReSTOR intraocular lens implants. *Am J Ophthalmol*. 2007;144(3):347-357.

19. Montes-Mico R, Espana E, Bueno I, Charman WN, Menezo JL. Visual performance with multifocal intraocular lenses: mesopic contrast sensitivity under distance and near conditions. *Ophthalmol.* 2004;111(1):85-96.

20. Martinez Palmer A, Gomez Faina P, Espana Albelda A, Comas Serrano M, Nahra Saad D, Castilla Cespedes M. Visual function with bilateral implantation of monofocal and multifocal intraocular lenses: a prospective, randomized, controlled clinical trial. *J Refract Surg.* 2008;24(3):257-264.

21. de Vries NE, Webers CA, Touwslager WR, et al. Dissatisfaction after implantation of multifocal intraocular lenses. *J Cataract Refract Surg.* 2011;37(5):859-865.

22. Solomon R, Donnenfeld ED, Perry HD. The effects of LASIK on the ocular surface. *Ocul Surf.* 2004;2(1):34-44.

23. Albietz JM, McLennan SG, Lenton LM. Ocular surface management of photorefractive keratectomy and laser in situ keratomileusis. *J Refract Surg.* 2003;19(6):636-644.

24. Toda I, Asano-Kato N, Hori-Komai Y, Tsubota K. Laser-assisted in situ keratomileusis for patients with dry eye. *Arch Ophthalmol.* 2002;120(8):1024-1028.

25. Eydelman M, Hilmantel G, Tarver ME, et al. Symptoms and Satisfaction of Patients in the Patient-Reported Outcomes With Laser In Situ Keratomileusis (PROWL) Studies. *JAMA Ophthalmol.* 2017;135(1):13-22.

26. Garcia-Zalisnak D, Nash D, Yeu E. Ocular surface diseases and corneal refractive surgery. *Curr Opin Ophthalmol.* 2014;25(4):264-269.

27. Fraunfelder FT, Fraunfelder FW, Edwards R. Ocular side effects possibly associated with isotretinoin usage. *Am J Ophthalmol.* 2001;132(3):299-305.

28. Mathers WD, Shields WJ, Sachdev MS, Petroll WM, Jester JV. Meibomian gland morphology and tear osmolarity: changes with Accutane therapy. *Cornea.* 1991;10(4):286-290.

29. Bragheeth MA, Dua HS. Corneal sensation after myopic and hyperopic LASIK: clinical and confocal microscopic study. *Br J Ophthalmol.* 2005;89(5):580-585.

30. Shoja MR, Besharati MR. Dry eye after LASIK for myopia: Incidence and risk factors. *Eur J Ophthalmol.* 2007;17(1):1-6.

31. Tuisku IS, Lindbohm N, Wilson SE, Tervo TM. Dry eye and corneal sensitivity after high myopic LASIK. *J Refract Surg.* 2007;23(4):338-342.

32. Whitcher JP, Shiboski CH, Shiboski SC, et al. A simplified quantitative method for assessing keratoconjunctivitis sicca from the sjogren's syndrome international registry. *Am J Ophthalmol.* 2010;149(3):405-415.

33. Raoof D, Pineda R. Dry eye after laser in-situ keratomileusis. *Semin Ophthalmol.* 2014;29(5-6):358-362.

34. Randleman JB, Woodward M, Lynn MJ, Stulting RD. Risk assessment for ectasia after corneal refractive surgery. *Ophthalmol.* 2008;115(1):37-50.

35. Tsai PS, Dowidar A, Naseri A, McLeod SD. Predicting time to refractive stability after discontinuation of rigid contact lens wear before refractive surgery. *J Cataract Refract Surg.* 2004;30(11):2290-2294.

36. 36.   Budak K, Hamed AM, Friedman NJ, Koch DD. Preoperative screening of contact lens wearers before refractive surgery. *J Cataract Refract Surg.* 1999;25(8):1080-1086.

37. de Paiva CS, Lindsey JL, Pflugfelder SC. Assessing the severity of keratitis sicca with videokeratoscopic indices. *Ophthalmol.* 2003;110(6):1102-1109.

38. De Paiva CS, Harris LD, Pflugfelder SC. Keratoconus-like topographic changes in keratoconjunctivitis sicca. *Cornea.* 2003;22(1):22-24.

39. Qin B, Chen S, Brass R, et al. Keratoconus diagnosis with optical coherence tomography-based pachymetric scoring system. *J Cataract Refract Surg.* 2013;39(12):1864-1871.

40. Ibrahim OM, Dogru M, Takano Y, et al. Application of visante optical coherence tomography tear meniscus height measurement in the diagnosis of dry eye disease. *Ophthalmol.* 2010;117(10):1923-1929.

41. Tung CI, Perin AF, Gumus K, Pflugfelder SC. Tear meniscus dimensions in tear dysfunction and their correlation with clinical parameters. *Am J Ophthalmol.* 2014;157(2):301-310.e301.

42. Alkharashi M, Lindsley K, Law HA, Sikder S. Medical interventions for acanthamoeba keratitis. *Cochrane Database Syst Rev.* 2015;2:Cd010792.

43. Tomlinson A, Khanal S, Ramaesh K, Diaper C, McFadyen A. Tear film osmolarity: determination of a referent for dry eye diagnosis. *Invest Ophthalmol Vis Sci.* 2006;47(10):4309-4315.

44. Amparo F, Hamrah P, Schaumberg DA, Dana R. The value of tear osmolarity as a metric in evaluating the response to dry eye therapy in the clinic and in clinical trials. *Am J Ophthalmol.* 2014;157(4):915-916.

45. Amparo F, Jin Y, Hamrah P, Schaumberg DA, Dana R. What is the value of incorporating tear osmolarity measurement in assessing patient response to therapy in dry eye disease? *Am J Ophthalmol.* 2014;157(1):69-77.e62.

46. Toda I, Asano-Kato N, Komai-Hori Y, Tsubota K. Dry eye after laser in situ keratomileusis. *Am J Ophthalmol.* 2001;132(1):1-7.

47. Alfawaz AM, Algehedan S, Jastaneiah SS, Al-Mansouri S, Mousa A, Al-Assiri A. Efficacy of punctal occlusion in management of dry eyes after laser in situ keratomileusis for myopia. *Curr Eye Res.* 2014;39(3):257-262.

48. Salib GM, McDonald MB, Smolek M. Safety and efficacy of cyclosporine 0.05% drops versus unpreserved artificial tears in dry-eye patients having laser in situ keratomileusis. *J Cataract Refract Surg.* 2006;32(5):772-778.

49. Hessert D, Tanzer D, Brunstetter T, Kaupp S, Murdoch D, Mirzaoff M. Topical cyclosporine A for postoperative photorefractive keratectomy and laser in situ keratomileusis. *J Cataract Refract Surg.* 2013;39(4):539-547.

50. Donnenfeld ED, Solomon R, Roberts CW, Wittpenn JR, McDonald MB, Perry HD. Cyclosporine 0.05% to improve visual outcomes after multifocal intraocular lens implantation. *J Cataract Refract Surg.* 2010;36(7):1095-1100.

51. Pucker AD, Ng SM, Nichols JJ. Over the counter (OTC) artificial tear drops for dry eye syndrome. *Cochrane Database Syst Rev.* 2016;2:Cd009729.

52. Sheppard JD, Jr., Singh R, McClellan AJ, et al. Long-term supplementation with n-6 and n-3 PUFAs improves moderate-to-severe keratoconjunctivitis sicca: a randomized double-blind clinical trial. *Cornea.* 2013;32(10):1297-1304.

53. Deinema LA, Vingrys AJ, Wong CY, Jackson DC, Chinnery HR, Downie LE. A randomized, double-masked, placebo-controlled clinical trial of two forms of omega-3 supplements for treating dry eye disease. *Ophthalmol.* 2017;124(1):43-52.

54. Liu A, Ji J. Omega-3 essential fatty acids therapy for dry eye syndrome: a meta-analysis of randomized controlled studies. *Med Sci Monit.* 2014;20:1583-1589.

55. Kawakita T, Kawabata F, Tsuji T, Kawashima M, Shimmura S, Tsubota K. Effects of dietary supplementation with fish oil on dry eye syndrome subjects: randomized controlled trial. *Biomed Res.* 2013;34(5):215-220.

56. Creuzot-Garcher C, Baudouin C, Labetoulle M, et al. [Efficacy assessment of Nutrilarm®, a per os omega-3 and omega-6 polyunsaturated essential fatty acid dietary formulation versus placebo in patients with bilateral treated moderate dry eye syndrome]. *J Fr Ophtalmol.* 2011;34(7):448-455.

57. De Paiva CS, Corrales RM, Villarreal AL, et al. Apical corneal barrier disruption in experimental murine dry eye is abrogated by methylprednisolone and doxycycline. *Invest Ophthalmol Vis Sci.* 2006;47(7):2847-2856.

58. Quarterman MJ, Johnson DW, Abele DC, Lesher JL, Jr., Hull DS, Davis LS. Ocular rosacea. Signs, symptoms, and tear studies before and after treatment with doxycycline. *Arch Dermatol.* 1997;133(1):49-54.

59. Yoo SE, Lee DC, Chang MH. The effect of low-dose doxycycline therapy in chronic meibomian gland dysfunction. *Korean J Ophthalmol.* 2005;19(4):258-263.

60. Xiao Q, Tan Y, Lin Z, et al. Minocycline inhibits inflammation and squamous metaplasia of conjunctival tissue culture in airlift conditions. *Cornea.* 2016;35(2):249-256.

61. Marsh P, Pflugfelder SC. Topical nonpreserved methylprednisolone therapy for keratoconjunctivitis sicca in Sjogren syndrome. *Ophthalmol.* 1999;106(4):811-816.

62. Pflugfelder SC, Maskin SL, Anderson B, et al. A randomized, double-masked, placebo-controlled, multicenter comparison of loteprednol etabonate ophthalmic suspension, 0.5%, and placebo for treatment of keratoconjunctivitis sicca in patients with delayed tear clearance. *Am J Ophthalmol.* 2004;138(3):444-457.

63. Jonisch J, Steiner A, Udell IJ. Preservative-free low-dose dexamethasone for the treatment of chronic ocular surface disease refractory to standard therapy. *Cornea.* 2010;29(7):723-726.

64. Avunduk AM, Avunduk MC, Varnell ED, Kaufman HE. The comparison of efficacies of topical corticosteroids and nonsteroidal anti-inflammatory drops on dry eye patients: a clinical and immunocytochemical study. *Am J Ophthalmol.* 2003;136(4):593-602.

65. Wan PX, Wang XR, Song YY, et al. Study on the treatment of dry eye with loteprednol etabonate. *Zhonghua Yan Ke Za Zhi.* 2012;48(2):142-147.

66. Sall K, Stevenson OD, Mundorf TK, Reis BL. Two multicenter, randomized studies of the efficacy and safety of cyclosporine ophthalmic emulsion in moderate to severe dry eye disease. CsA Phase 3 Study Group. *Ophthalmol.* 2000;107(4):631-639.

67. Rao SN. Topical cyclosporine 0.05% for the prevention of dry eye disease progression. *J Ocul Pharmacol Ther.* 2010;26(2):157-164.

68. Pflugfelder SC, De Paiva CS, Villarreal AL, Stern ME. Effects of sequential artificial tear and cyclosporine emulsion therapy on conjunctival goblet cell density and transforming growth factor-beta2 production. *Cornea.* 2008;27(1):64-69.

69. Holland EJ, Luchs J, Karpecki PM, et al. Lifitegrast for the treatment of dry eye disease: results of a Phase III, randomized, double-masked, placebo-controlled trial (OPUS-3). *Ophthalmol.* 2017;124(1):53-60.

70. Holland EJ, Whitley WO, Sall K, et al. Lifitegrast clinical efficacy for treatment of signs and symptoms of dry eye disease across three randomized controlled trials. *Curr Med Res Opin.* 2016;22:1-7.

71. Sheppard JD, Torkildsen GL, Lonsdale JD, et al. Lifitegrast ophthalmic solution 5.0% for treatment of dry eye disease: results of the OPUS-1 phase 3 study. *Ophthalmol.* 2014;121(2):475-483.

72. Tauber J, Karpecki P, Latkany R, et al. Lifitegrast ophthalmic solution 5.0% versus placebo for treatment of dry eye disease: results of the randomized Phase III OPUS-2 study. *Ophthalmol.* 2015;122(12):2423-2431.

CHAPTER 15

What Is Your Treatment Paradigm?

PART 1

Ashley R. Brissette MD, MSc, FRCSC and
Christopher E. Starr, MD

KEY POINTS

- Signs and symptoms of dry eye disease (DED) may not correlate.
- Tear osmolarity and matrix metalloproteinase-9 (MMP-9) testing are noninvasive, quick, simple, point-of-care diagnostic tests.
- Meibography and thermal pulsation are more recent additions to the treatment paradigm.

The approach to the diagnosis and treatment of dry eye disease (DED) has changed considerably over the past number of years. This is largely due to a better understanding of the pathophysiology of this complex disease. Often multifactorial, DED can be difficult to diagnose and manage. However, the availability of diagnostic testing, as well

Mah FS, Rhee MK, eds.
Dry Eye Disease: A Practical Guide (pp 155-186).
© 2019 Taylor & Francis Group.

as an increase in the number of treatment modalities, has changed the face of DED over the years. What used to exist as an entity that most clinicians preferred to avoid, DED is now at the forefront of many ophthalmology practices. The sheer volume of publications on DED has increased exponentially, and is a trend that does not seem to be slowing down.[1] The available approved diagnostic testing for DED has also increased in recent times, which has furthered our ability to properly diagnose this complex condition. Although DED is often thought of as a singular condition, we prefer to consider it as one component within a broad category of many ocular surface diseases (OSDs). By refining the terminology to encompass both DED and OSD together, we are better able to direct our diagnostic and treatment protocols to include all potential causes of patient symptoms. A systematic algorithmic approach to diagnosing the underlying pathophysiologic components of DED/OSD is the key to our diagnostic protocol and treatment paradigm.

The foundation of our current approach to DED/OSD is largely based on the 2007 report of the International Dry Eye WorkShop (DEWS).[2] We anxiously awaited the update to this report, which was published 10 years after the first edition in 2017. The 2017 International Dry Eye WorkShop (DEWS II) is the most up-to-date, comprehensive report on DED/OSD.[3] Our treatment protocol was developed around the definition of DED, as this is an important factor in understanding the disease process. Both the original DEWS and the DEWS II incorporate hyperosmolarity and ocular surface inflammation and damage into the definition of DED.[2,3] The importance of recognizing inflammation as a key factor in the underlying pathophysiology of DED/OSD cannot be understated. In fact, a systematic review of the literature found that many studies have supported the core role of inflammation in the pathophysiologic process of DED.[1] As such, identifying and treating this underlying inflammation plays an important role in our treatment paradigm. Given the breadth of research establishing inflammation as a key factor in DED/OSD, we believe that inflammation should be identified and treated in the early stages of the disease. If ignored, the inflammation and associated inflammatory damage can worsen over time, impacting treatment efficacy, patient comfort, and even quality of life.

The first step in our, and most other, treatment protocols is identifying symptomatic patients. The Ocular Surface Disease Index (OSDI), Symptoms Assessment in Dry Eye (SANDE), or Standard Patient Evaluation of Eye Dryness (SPEED) are just a few examples of validated questionnaires that may be used in a clinical setting to identify symptomatic patients.[4-6] These questionnaires can be provided to the patient upon arrival to the clinic, or beforehand via the Internet, and then reviewed by an ophthalmic technician or similar first-line staff member. Outside of research, we would argue that written questionnaires for all patients is not mandatory, as well-trained technicians can (and should) verbally educe characteristic symptoms of DED/OSD during the initial history of present illness. Common symptoms elicited by our technicians are fluctuating vision, reduced visual quality, foreign body sensation, ocular discomfort, itching, photophobia, conjunctival injection, eyelid crusting, and computer-related ocular discomfort amongst others. If the patient confirms any symptoms suggestive of DED, then the technician proceeds with a careful history taking, focusing on exposure to risk factors for DED/OSD (ie, prior ocular diagnoses and surgeries, concurrent medications

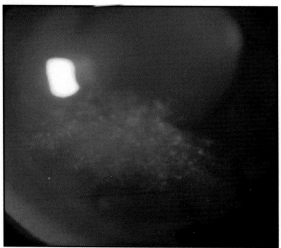

Figure 15-1. Significant inferior punctate epithelial erosions are noted on slit-lamp examination with cobalt blue light. The patient was asymptomatic, illustrating that signs and symptoms of DED may be poorly correlated.

that can exacerbate DED, contact lens wear and comfort, artificial tear use, comorbid autoimmune and dermatologic conditions and symptoms, etc). As per our protocol, when any DED/OSD-related symptom is identified, and after careful documentation of the ocular and systemic history, our technicians then proceed to point-of-care, in-office testing for DED/OSD. These tests are performed before the ocular surface milieu can be iatrogenically altered by the eye exam or instillation of any drops.

Although these questionnaires and interrogations are useful in identifying patients with DED symptoms, research and experience has shown that subjective symptoms do not always correlate well with clinical objective measures of DED severity.[7] The disparity between signs and symptoms of DED can prove challenging in both establishing a diagnosis and effectively treating this common condition (Figure 15-1). One study which elucidates this concept is the Prospective Health Assessment of Cataract Patient Ocular Surface (PHACO) which demonstrated that 64% of preoperative cataract patients had an abnormal tear break-up time (TBUT), 77% of eyes had abnormal corneal fluorescein staining, while only 13% reported significant DED symptoms.[8] Our research team at Weill Cornell Medicine conducted a similar study evaluating the prevalence of abnormal point-of-care tear testing in minimally symptomatic to asymptomatic patients precataract surgery. We found that 75% had abnormal matrix metalloproteinase-9 (MMP-9) testing, 45% had abnormal tear osmolarity, and 40% were abnormal on both tests.[9] Therefore, we strongly recommend screening all preoperative refractive surgery patients (cataract, laser vision correction, etc) for DED/OSD despite the presence or absence of symptoms. The importance of the ocular surface on refractive outcomes cannot be understated, and oversight in diagnosing DED/OSD preop can result in poor visual outcomes. It has been demonstrated that in patients with abnormal tear osmolarity, there is significantly more variability in average keratometry readings and anterior corneal astigmatism with significant differences in intraocular lens power calculations of up to or above 0.5 D.[10] This concept highlights the importance of tear testing and careful clinical examination of all preoperative patients despite symptomatology, and

Figure 15-2. Tear osmolarity testing is a noninvasive, quick and simple point-of-care, in-office diagnostic test.

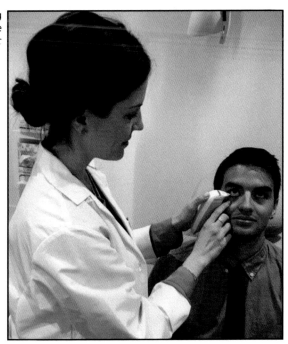

therefore, our protocol incorporates tear testing for all preoperative surgical patients (cataract or refractive).

In our practice, once DED symptoms are identified, the technician then performs tear osmolarity (TearLab Osmolarity System, TearLab) and tear MMP-9 testing (InflammaDry, Quidel). These are noninvasive, quick and simple point-of-care, in-office diagnostic tests (Figure 15-2). Tear osmolarity testing has been established as a useful tool in the diagnosis and staging of DED across many studies.[11-13] In fact, a recent review of the literature found a 72% positive impression of tear osmolarity testing in establishing a DED diagnosis.[14] This type of testing offers an objective quantitative value for classifying results.[15] An osmolarity of 308 mOsm/L or greater, or an inter-eye difference (signifying tear film instability) of 8 mOsm/L or greater, is significant for establishing a diagnosis of DED, and this value is linearly related to severity of DED (320 mOsm/L or greater = moderate DED, 330 mOsm/L or greater = severe DED). Tear testing is then repeated at follow-up visits, as serial osmolarity testing is useful for gauging treatment efficacy and guiding treatment decisions.

MMP-9 is an inflammatory mediator released by distressed epithelial cells.[16-18] The level of MMP-9 is elevated in the tear film in DED and also some other types of OSD. When compared to a combination of routine clinical dry eye diagnostic criteria, it demonstrated a sensitivity of 85% and a specificity of 94%.[19] When both the tear osmolarity and MMP-9 tests are abnormal in a symptomatic patient, it suggests a diagnosis of DED with significant ocular surface inflammation. Our treatment plan will include anti-inflammatory medications in addition to other DED therapies. When the tear osmolarity is abnormal but the MMP-9 is normal, it suggests to us a diagnosis

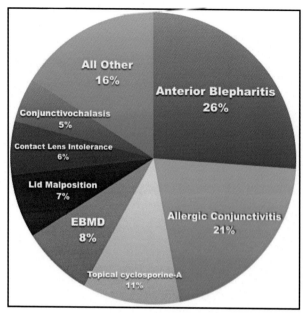

Figure 15-3. The most commonly diagnosed ocular conditions found in patients with DED-like symptoms and normal tear osmolarity testing.

of DED without significant inflammation and thus anti-inflammatory medications might not be indicated. The scenario of normal osmolarity and elevated MMP-9, in the context of ocular surface symptoms, suggests a possible diagnosis of a non-dry eye ocular surface disorder (NDEOSD). A study by our research group evaluated 100 consecutive symptomatic patients with normal tear osmolarity and determined that the most common causes for DED-like symptoms were allergic conjunctivitis (26%), anterior blepharitis (21%), treatment with topical cyclosporine A (CsA) 0.05% (11%), and epithelial basement membrane dystrophy (8%), and eyelid malpositions (7%) including lagophthalmos and floppy eyelid syndrome (Figure 15-3)[19]. Lastly, when both tear tests are normal, potential causes for the patient's symptoms may include incipient or situational DED (computer vision syndrome, low humidity, etc) keratoneuralgia ("pain without stain" or neuropathic pain syndrome) and compensated or treated DED. It should be emphasized that utilizing point-of-care diagnostic testing does not, and never will, replace a careful slit-lamp exam and clinician acumen, and when DED is advanced and obvious, the diagnostic utility of these tests is less useful. Still, we find tremendous benefit from these tests in the less obvious, subtler cases of DED and for identifying DED masqueraders. Other diagnostic tests such as tear IgE, tear lactoferrin, Sjögren syndrome testing, among others, in conjunction with those discussed above, may also help differentiate the underlying cause of ocular surface symptoms and thereby further increase diagnostic accuracy.

Although osmolarity and MMP-9 testing are useful in ruling in, or out, a diagnosis of DED, they are unable to distinguish between the 2 most common subtypes of DED: evaporative dry eye disease (EDED) and aqueous-deficient dry eye disease (ADDED). Therefore, the next step in our treatment protocol after determining the presence of DED is determining the subtype to tailor our treatment regimen. Although the

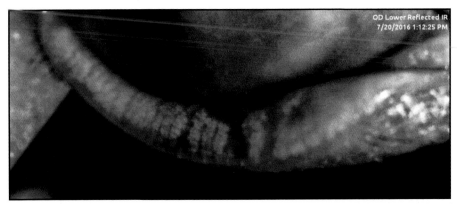

Figure 15-4. High-resolution meibomian gland imaging (meibography) showing gland dropout and atrophy from meibomian gland dysfunction.

classification describes 2 distinct subtypes, patients often have an overlap or 'mixed' form of DED. A careful slit-lamp examination should be performed, including objective measures such as TBUT, tear meniscus height, examination and expression of the meibomian glands, eyelid position, blink quality, and vital dye staining of the cornea and conjunctiva. Schirmer or phenol red thread testing can be performed to assess tear production. These tests can further delineate the underlying pathophysiologic process most responsible for the patient's symptoms. Of note, if the exam, symptoms and/or test results suggest a primarily aqueous-deficient DED, we recommend a systemic work-up to rule out Sjögren syndrome in those patients with characteristic symptoms. Traditional blood tests and/or referral to a rheumatologist are reasonable as is performing the more convenient point-of-care finger-stick blood test (Sjö, Bausch + Lomb) within the ophthalmic office setting.

Newer diagnostic tests may also help differentiate between aqueous and evaporative DED. If there is evidence of meibomian gland dysfunction (MGD) at the slit-lamp (or presence of it on history) we perform meibomian gland imaging. This allows us to assess the presence and severity of MGD and also helps with classification towards EDED or mixed type DED. The LipiView & LipiScan machines (TearScience) provide high-resolution imaging of the meibomian glands (meibography), which provides information on the morphology and health of the meibomian glands, along with analysis of the blink quality and lipid layer thickness (Figure 15-4).[20] The OCULUS Keratograph 5M (OCULUS) can also image the meibomian glands, as well as provide noninvasive TBUT and tear meniscus height measurement, as well as objectively grade eye redness. Other imaging modalities such as in vivo confocal microscopy can reveal meibomian gland dropout and periglandular inflammation in chronic obstructive meibomian gland disease.[21] Optical coherence tomography (OCT) can provide an objective value of tear meniscus height and area that, when low, is suggestive of an aqueous deficient DED, as is an abnormally low level of the lacrimal gland derived tear protein, lactoferrin.[22] Aberrometry and topography are other useful diagnostics for evaluating the interblink integrity of the tear film and may prove especially useful in laser vision correction screening.[23]

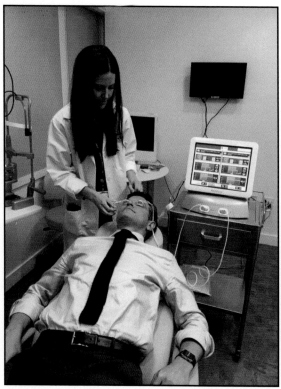

Figure 15-5. Thermal pulsation treatment to remove blockages from the meibomian glands can be performed in the office setting and may be of benefit for the treatment of EDED.

Once DED/OSD is effectively ruled in, and the subtype is determined, the treatment can be tailored specifically to the patient. Although beyond the scope of this chapter, our treatment protocol is tightly linked to the results of the above diagnostic work-up. In DED patients, we carefully select a multipronged treatment regimen based on the severity, the presence or absence of inflammation, and the underlying etiology and predominant DED subtype, all of which are established by the diagnostic algorithm. When the subtype is primarily aqueous deficient, environmental modifications, tear supplements, topical anti-inflammatories and/or punctal occlusion are reasonable options. If primarily evaporative DED, nutritional supplements, eyelid care (scrubs, warm compresses, massage, etc) topical or oral antibiotics, topical anti-inflammatories and various procedures (thermal pulsation, blepharoexfoliation, meibomian gland probing, etc) can be of benefit (Figure 15-5). Mixed aqueous deficient and evaporative DED/OSD will benefit from a multifactorial approach to treatment, and newer neurostimulation devices, such as the TrueTear device (Allergan), may prove useful in these cases. After instituting treatment, follow-up visits should include repeating all components of the protocol including the symptoms questionnaire, tear testing, imaging, other available ancillary tests and a careful slit-lamp examination. Repeating the above protocol is essential to monitor the efficacy of the treatment regimen and to make changes that are tailored to the patient's outcome.

Summary

As illustrated previously, our current treatment paradigm begins with identifying symptomatic patients via questionnaires or technician directed questions to elicit symptoms of potential DED/OSD. If such symptoms are determined, patients then undergo objective point-of-care diagnostic tear tests, initially including tear osmolarity and MMP-9. However, we strongly recommend that all patients seeking any form of refractive and cataract surgery undergo tear testing and further examination for DED/OSD regardless of symptomatology. If the combination of symptoms and technician performed tear testing suggests DED/OSD, further testing to differentiate between EDED and ADDED can be performed (meibography, tear OCT, lactoferrin, etc) followed by a careful slit-lamp examination. Since symptoms of multiple ocular surface disorders often overlap and are nonspecific, the above diagnostic algorithm and basket of test results will frequently lead to diagnoses of NDEOSDs or masqueraders. Whether a subtype of DED is diagnosed or another form of OSD is detected, a customized treatment regimen, based on disease severity, can be constructed for each patient. In order to monitor the treatment efficacy, subsequent examinations should include repeating the diagnostic algorithm and adjusting treatments based on the evolution of patient symptoms, test results, and clinical findings.

References

1. Wei Y, Asbell PA. The core mechanism of dry eye disease is inflammation. *Eye Contact Lens.* 2014;40(4):248-256.
2. The definition and classification of dry eye disease: report of the Definition and Classification Subcommittee of the International Dry Eye WorkShop (2007). *Ocul Surf.* 2007;5(2):75-92.
3. Craig J, Nichols K, Akpek E, et al. TFOS DEWS II definition and classification report. *Ocul Surf.* 2017;15(3):276-283.
4. Ngo W, Situ P, Keir N, Korb D, Blackie C, Simpson T. Psychometric properties and validation of the standard patient evaluation of eye dryness questionnaire. *Cornea.* 2013;32(9):1204-1210.
5. Schiffman RM, Christianson MD, Jacobsen G, Hirsch JD, Reis BL. Reliability and validity of the ocular surface disease index. *Arch Ophthalmol.* 2000;118(5):615-621.
6. Schaumberg DA, Gulati A, Mathers WD, et al. Development and validation of a short global dry eye symptom index. *Ocul Surf.* 2007;5(1):50-57.
7. Nichols KK, Nichols JJ, Mitchell GL. The lack of association between signs and symptoms in patients with dry eye disease. *Cornea.* 2004;23(8):762-770.
8. Trattler WB, Majmudar PA, Donnenfeld ED, McDonald MB, Stonecipher KG, Goldberg DF. The prospective health assessment of cataract patients' ocular surface (PHACO) study: the effect of dry eye. *Clin Ophthalmol.* 2017;11:1423-1430.
9. Gupta PK, Drinkwater OJ, VanDusen KW, Brissette AR, Starr CE. Prevalence of ocular surface dysfunction in patients presenting for cataract surgery evaluation. *J Cataract Refract Surg.* 2018;44(9):1090-1096.
10. Epitropoulos AT, Matossian C, Berdy GJ, Malhotra RP, Potvin R. Effect of tear osmolarity on repeatability of keratometry for cataract surgery planning. *J Cataract Refract Surg.* 2015;41(8):1672-1677.
11. Lemp MA. Advances in understanding and managing dry eye disease. *Am J Ophthalmol.* 2008;146(3):350-356.
12. Lemp MA, Bron AJ, Baudouin C, et al. Tear osmolarity in the diagnosis and management of dry eye disease. *Am J Ophthalmol.* 2011;151(5):792-798.e1.

13. Liu H, Begley C, Chen M, et al. A link between tear instability and hyperosmolarity in dry eye. *Invest Ophthalmol Vis Sci*. 2009;50(8):3671-3679.

14. Potvin R, Makari S, Rapuano CJ. Tear film osmolarity and dry eye disease: A review of the literature. *Clin Ophthalmol*. 2015;9:2039-2047.

15. Benelli U, Nardi M, Posarelli C, Albert TG. Tear osmolarity measurement using the TearLab osmolarity system in the assessment of dry eye treatment effectiveness. *Cont Lens Anterior Eye*. 2010;33(2):61-67.

16. Solomon A, Dursun D, Liu Z, Xie Y, Macri A, Pflugfelder SC. Pro- and anti-inflammatory forms of interleukin-1 in the tear fluid and conjunctiva of patients with dry-eye disease. *Invest Ophthalmol Vis Sci*. 2001;42(10):2283-2292.

17. Chotikavanich S, de Paiva CS, Li DQ, et al. Production and activity of matrix metalloproteinase-9 on the ocular surface increase in dysfunctional tear syndrome. *Invest Ophthalmol Vis Sci*. 2009;50(7):3203-3209.

18. Luo L, Li D, Doshi A, Farley W, Corrales RM, Pflugfelder SC. Experimental dry eye stimulates production of inflammatory cytokines and MMP-9 and activates MAPK signaling pathways on the ocular surface. *Invest Ophthalmol Vis Sci*. 2004;45(12):4293-4301.

19. Sambursky R, Davitt WF3, Latkany R, et al. Sensitivity and specificity of a point-of-care matrix metalloproteinase 9 immunoassay for diagnosing inflammation related to dry eye. *JAMA Ophthalmol*. 2013;131(1):24-28.

20. Blackie CA, Solomon JD, Scaffidi RC, Greiner JV, Lemp MA, Korb DR. The relationship between dry eye symptoms and lipid layer thickness. *Cornea*. 2009;28(7):789-794.

21. Ibrahim OMA, Matsumoto Y, Dogru M, et al. In vivo confocal microscopy evaluation of meibomian gland dysfunction in atopic-keratoconjunctivitis patients. *Ophthalmology*. 2012;119(10):1961-1968.

22. Shen M, Li J, Wang J, et al. Upper and lower tear menisci in the diagnosis of dry eye. *Invest Ophthalmol Vis Sci*. 2009;50(6):2722-2726.

23. Wang Y, Xu J, Sun X, Chu R, Zhuang H, He JC. Dynamic wavefront aberrations and visual acuity in normal and dry eyes. *Clin Exp Optom*. 2009;92(3):267-273.

PART 2

Walt Whitley, OD, MBA and John Sheppard, MD, MMSc

KEY POINTS

◆ A step-wise treatment based on severity levels of dry eye include: tear supplementation, eyelid hygiene, anti-inflammatory therapy, punctual plugs, oral antibiotics, thermal pulsation, and amniotic membrane (AM).

◆ Point-of-care testing to guide treatment includes: tear osmolarity, MMP-9, and dynamic meibography.

The treatment for DED continues to evolve as we gain more understanding of the disease, contributing factors, underlying causes, and current and emerging treatment options. Consensus guidelines have provided treatment recommendations based on severity levels with several additions to the paradigm. Point-of-care testing has provided additional objective data to justify appropriate initial treatment as well as chronic disease management. From tear supplements to nutraceuticals to meibomian gland and anti-inflammatory therapies, treatments are based according to the severity levels in which patients present for both initial and long-term therapy. The treatments presented in this chapter will provide an evidence-based rationale to addressing this chronic, progressive disease.

CHANGE IN PHILOSOPHY IN DRY EYE MANAGEMENT

The decision to treat patients who suffer from DED has significantly changed over the years. From the International Task Force Delphi panel recommendations, DEWS, and the International Workshop on Meibomian Gland Dysfunction, our understanding of dry eye treatments has seen rapid improvement.[1-4] With the increased awareness that MGD may well be the leading cause of DED throughout the world, there has been a shift in the treatment paradigm.[3] When addressing patients with dry eye, it is critical to identify and treat the underlying cause or causes of dry eye, to prioritize treatment accordingly, and decipher outcomes analytically rather than intuitively. In addition, measuring and managing the sequelae of the disease demand attention. Identification and differentiation of the classic OSD triad of MGD, lacrimal gland dysfunction, and allergy in each patient is necessary to treat appropriately. Regardless of the cause of DED, a combination of proactive treatment therapies may be necessary to reestablish a healthy ocular surface and treat the underlying cause early on in the disease state.

TREATMENT BASED ON CLINICAL SITUATION

Three general scenarios present to clinicians who recognize and treat dry eye.

1. *A new patient, often referred, presenting for the treatment of dry eye, usually having seen one or more previous providers and tried several unsuccessful treatments.* This patient requires a careful diagnostic evaluation with a step wise, logical, scientific introduction of 1 therapy at a time, and allowing adequate time for full treatment effect (at least 6 weeks). It can be useful to introduce 1 rapid onset therapy, such as topical steroids or punctal plugs, plus 1 slower onset therapy, such as nutritionals, eyelid scrubs or thermal pulsation, thereby allowing both the patient and clinician to differentiate between the 2 interventions.

2. *An existing patient with another primary diagnosis who is identified with dry eye.* Careful introduction of new treatments is again warranted, with careful attention to minimizing excessive drop use, particularly in glaucoma patients. These clinic visits may require more than the usual visit time due to their complexity, so the temptation to shrug off significant punctate keratopathy or increased discomfort until the next visit should be suppressed. Some patients with obvious ocular surface damage experience minimal discomfort and require more thorough explanations and intensive encouragement.

3. *A new or existing patient preparing for surgery.* Meticulous attention must always be paid to the condition of the refractive surface in order to optimize biometry,

healing, and surgical outcomes. In this situation, expeditious ocular surface normalization is preferred so multiple complementary therapies may be simultaneously initiated. Many of our cataract, corneal refractive, glaucoma, retina, oculoplastic, and transplant patients receive an immediate recommendation for all or most of the following to hasten response time: oral nutritionals, preservative free tears, eyelid scrubs containing hypochlorous acid (Avenova, NovaBay Pharmaceuticals; Hypochlor, OCuSOFT), punctal plugs, oral doxycycline, thermal pulsation, and topical loteprednol (Lotemax, Bausch + Lomb), CsA (Restasis, Allergan) or lifitegrast 5% (Xiidra, Shire).

Thus, patient-centered recommendations reflect the urgency, etiology, and severity of each clinical presentation.

TREATMENT BASED ON SEVERITY LEVELS

There have been several consensus guidelines which offer therapeutic guidelines based on the severity of the disease. In 2006, the Delphi Panel coined the term *dysfunctional tear syndrome* (DTS) which may present as DTS with eyelid margin disease, DTS with abnormal tear distribution, and DTS without eyelid margin disease. The latter was presented then as the most common form with treatment recommendations based on severity levels. Instead of relying primarily on currently available objective tests at the time, the panel recommended basing decisions mainly on patient signs and symptoms, including the presence or absence of eyelid margin disease and tear distribution anomalies, as well as on the severity of the disease as defined by multiple suggested criteria. With more advanced disease, additional treatment options may become necessary.[1]

In 2007, members of the management and treatment subcommittee of the DEWS followed many of the conventions established by the Delphi panel, adding additional criteria, more specific signs and symptoms for each of the Delphi panel's 4 levels of severity, as well as additional ancillary treatment recommendations that were not included in the International Task Force guidelines. These recommendations may be modified by practitioners based on individual patient profiles and clinical experience.[2]

In 2011, MGD came into the forefront of clinical research and clinical care with the MGD report. The MGD report has been utilized in a similar fashion to the DEWS report, providing an evidence-based approach to the management of MGD. At each treatment level, lack of response to therapy moves treatment to the next level.[3]

In 2017, the DEWS II report was published. The DEWS II defined dry eye as "a multifactorial disease of the ocular surface characterized by a loss of homeostasis of the tear film, and accompanied by ocular symptoms, in which tear film instability and hyperosmolarity, ocular surface inflammation and damage, and neurosensory abnormalities play etiological roles."[3]

With the plethora of research and evidence-based literature available corroborating these reports, the current treatment paradigm should be modified by each practitioner based on the presentation. Unfortunately, patients who present with dry eye do not often occupy individual silos of either aqueous deficient or evaporative dry eye, with or without the influence of allergic disease, so a combination of treatments is warranted. Proper diagnosis of all forms of DED will determine the appropriate treatment based on severity level.

STAGE 1 DRY EYE DISEASE (AQUEOUS +/- EVAPORATIVE DEFICIENT)

Patient education is tantamount: understanding contributory factors, including environment, systemic and topical medications, allergy control and the presence of MGD. Tear supplementation remains the primary treatment. Key concerns in the selection of an artifical tear include the role of preservatives, the role of viscosity, and more recently, the supplementation of oil (lipid) to the tear film. Another consideration is eyelid hygiene including warm compresses, cleansing with hypochlorous acid scrub preparations, and expression of the meibomian glands.

TEAR SUPPLEMENTATION

Lubricating eye drops or "artificial tears" are a traditional mainstay in the treatment of DED, yet patients have sought relief either directly from the pharmacy, recommendation by a friend or family member, or random preference from the over-the-counter shelf before ever seeking a prescription from their eye care provider (ECP). Although tear supplements may provide temporary relief, they do not adequately address the underlying cause of either aqueous deficient or evaporative disease. Often, patients have tried numerous artificial tears or topical vasoconstrictors prior to seeking professional treatment. Tear selection can be titrated to patient preferences and the ECP evaluation, but there has been no large scale, masked, comparative clinical trials to evaluate the wide variety of ocular lubricants.

EYELID HYGIENE

Eyelid hygiene is a mainstay of treatment which consists of a combination of 45°C heat, eyelid scrubs, and expression. Warm compresses are commonly recommended with a continuous application for at least 4 minutes with optimal contact between compress and eyelid, replacing the compress every 2 minutes with a new preheated compress. Eyelid expression techniques vary from gentle massage of the eyelids against the eyeball to forceful squeezing of the eyelids either directly or against each other to address MGD.[5] Excessive colonization of the eyelid margin can be controlled with commercial eyelid wipes (Avenova, NovaBay Pharmaceuticals; Hypochlor, OCuSOFT) or the traditional diluted baby shampoo.[6]

STAGE 2 DRY EYE DISEASE
(AQUEOUS +/- EVAPORATIVE DEFICIENT)

Patients who present with moderate DED signs and symptoms warrant Stage 1 treatment plus anti-inflammatory and antibiotic medications. More viscous tear supplements or preservative-free formulations and ointments may be necessary. With or without obvious inflammatory signs, topical steroids, CsA, lifitegrast 5%, and nutraceuticals provide proactive control of otherwise progressive inflammatory ocular surface damage. If moderate MGD is present, topical or systemic antibiotics may be utilized. Temporary collagen or silicone punctal occlusion is also recommended at this stage.

ANTI-INFLAMMATORY THERAPY

Anti-inflammatory therapy has become a mainstay of treatment. Corticosteroids are an effective anti-inflammatory therapy in both acute and chronic DED. In a 4-week, double-masked, randomized study in 64 patients with keratoconjunctivitis sicca and delayed tear clearance, loteprednol etabonate 0.5% ophthalmic suspension (Lotemax, Bausch + Lomb) 4 times a day, was found to be more effective than its vehicle in improving some signs and symptoms.[7] Topical CsA boasts a 13-year track record as a safe and effective treatment for dry eye. In clinical studies, CsA is believed to inhibit T-cell activation, decrease tear cytokines, and increase goblet cell density.[8] Additionally, the vehicle for CsA consists of castor oil which targets the lipid layer of the tears. Corticosteroids may also be considered for induction therapy 2 weeks before the initiation of long-term CsA treatment for chronic DED to provide more rapid relief of dry eye signs and symptoms with greater efficacy than CsA and artifical tear alone.[9]

The addition of lifitegrast 5% to the market has become a welcome addition to our current treatments. Lifitegrast 5% is a lymphocyte function-associated antigen-1 antagonist indicated for the treatment of the signs and symptoms of DED.[10]

For patients that present with MGD alone or combined aqueous deficiency, a consideration of either CsA or topical azithromycin may be warranted. In a non-inferiority study comparing a combination of tobramycin and dexamethasone vs CsA alone, improvements in Schirmer scores, TBUT, meibomian gland secretion, and symptoms were seen.[11] Another single-center trial evaluating topical 1% azithromycin solution demonstrated significant improvement in signs and symptoms of MGD after 2 and 4 weeks of treatment. Resolution of signs and symptoms correlated with spectroscopic analysis of expressed meibum, which demonstrated improvement in ordering of lipids and phase transition temperature of lipids in the meibomian gland secretion.[12]

Nutraceuticals play a significant role for patients with moderate to severe disease. Because MGD is associated with altered lipid composition, dietary supplementation with omega-3 fatty acids has been recommended in both the DEWS and International Workshop on Meibomian Gland Dysfunction as primary therapy.[2-3] In a multicenter, double-blind, randomized, placebo-controlled clinical trial, daily dietary supplementation with a unique combination of polyunsaturated fatty acids (Gamma-linolenic,

Eicosapentaenoic, and Docosahexaenoic) for 6 months is effective in improving ocular irritation symptoms and halting the progression of inflammation that characterizes moderate to severe dry eye.[13] In another study, a placebo-controlled, double-masked, randomized trial successfully measured supplement driven improvements in various endpoints including tear osmolarity, OSDI, TBUT, corneal staining, and omega-3 index levels.[14]

PUNCTAL PLUGS

Punctal plugs serve the purpose of occluding the tear drainage system by blocking tear drainage through the canaliculi. In doing so, they increase tear fluid accumulation, thereby keeping the ocular surface lubricated. Plugs provide instantaneous and long-term relief, reducing the need for frequent artificial tear use. Although often underutilized, beneficial outcome in dry eye symptoms has been reported in 74% to 86% of patients treated with punctal plugs.[15] Objective indices of improvement reported with the use of punctal plugs include improved corneal staining, prolonged TBUT, decrease in tear osmolarity, and increase in goblet cell density.[16] Punctal plugs do not directly address underlying ocular surface inflammation in DED so there is a need for concomitant anti-inflammatory therapy.

STAGES 3 AND 4 DRY EYE DISEASE (AQUEOUS +/- EVAPORATIVE DEFICIENT)

For more advanced signs and symptoms, additional treatments augment previous interventions. Often this may include a combination of topical anti-inflammatories as well as oral antibiotics. Additional treatment options may include autologous serum, topical Vitamin A, bandage contact lenses, amniotic membrane (AM) application, scleral contact lenses, moisture goggles, and surgery.[1-3]

ORAL ANTIBIOTICS

Patients with more advanced DED in either form may benefit from oral antibiotics. The tetracycline class has been the most commonly prescribed due to simultaneous antibacterial and anti-inflammatory properties. More recently, topical azithromycin has been shown to be as effective as oral doxycycline with a better effect on improving signs, better overall clinical response, and shorter duration of treatment.[17]

INNOVATIVE DRY EYE TREATMENT OPTIONS FOR MODERATE TO SEVERE CONDITIONS

Thermal Pulsation

The treatment of meibomian gland obstruction has become more commonly utilized for DED patients. LipiFlow (TearScience) received US Food and Drug Administration (FDA) clearance based on an open-label, randomized, controlled, multicenter trial.[18] A single-dose session offers the same efficacy profile as warm compresses while improving meibomian gland function and other correlates of ocular surface health.[19]

Amniotic Membranes

Human AM has been shown to provide a substantial benefit in treating numerous conjunctival and corneal diseases. For ocular surface conditions not responding to previous intervention, amniotic membranes provide a viable alternative used concurrently with other medications. Innate properties of AM include growth factors, collagen, fibronectin, and laminin, which promote regenerative healing. Additionally, AM has anti-inflammatory, antimicrobial, anti-angiogenic, and anti-scarring properties which may improve ocular surface health.[20-21] AM is available in cryopreserved and freeze-dried formats, and can be surgically sutured or glued into position, secured under a bandage contact lenes, or placed on the ocular surface as a sutureless trampoline device, such as the PROKERA (Bio-Tissue).

UTILIZATION OF POINT-OF-CARE TESTING TO GUIDE TREATMENT

Osmolarity

Tear osmolarity is a physiologic marker that can be used to understand and monitor tear film health and stability. Abnormal osmolarity indicates an unstable tear film, which can potentially damage the ocular surface and cornea. Tear osmolarity increases due to a decrease in aqueous production and/or a decrease in lipid production resulting in increased evaporation. According to Lemp et al, tear osmolarity is the most useful single objective test to differentiate those with early-stage mild or moderate dry eye from those with severe disease.[22] A cutoff threshold of more than 308 mOsms/L was found to be very sensitive in differentiating normal from mild to moderate subjects. Additionally, an inter-eye difference greater than 8 mOsm/L also indicates that the tear film is not in homeostasis, portending eventual ocular surface damage.

Tear osmolarity can be utilized to manage the therapeutic response to selected treatment. Several studies have demonstrated improvement in lowering tear film osmolarity to homeostatic levels using CsA, lubricants with hydroxypropyl guar, and nutritional supplements. If a therapy is effective, one should see a drop in osmolarity.[14,23-24]

Matrix Metalloproteinase-9

MMPs are proteolytic enzymes produced by stressed epithelial cells on the ocular surface. Although MMP-9 is a nonspecific inflammatory marker, OSD demonstrates elevated tear levels of MMP-9. Identifying elevated levels of MMP-9 facilitates better management of patients who present with signs or symptoms of DED. Patients who test positive can be treated with topical or oral anti-inflammatory medications such as steroids, CsA, lifitegrast 5%, azithromycin or doxycycline.[25-26]

Dynamic Meibography

Imaging of the inferior tarsal plate produces useful clinical data for the ECP, as well as understandable photographic motivation for patients. The ability to create serial semi-quantitative assessments of remaining functional meibomian glands provides practical information for treatment recommendations.

Strategic Analysis and Evidence-Based Medicine

Careful physical examination and thorough history documentation coupled with objective point of service testing yields a logical treatment selection best suited for a patient's most significant aberrations. This strategy should provide rapid clinical results, decreased use of random medications, fewer missed work days, longer efficient work hours unencumbered by dry eye symptoms, fewer return visits to the clinic, subsequently deceased travel miles, and thereby significantly lower overall health care costs to society.

Thus, the treatment paradigm is directed by each individual patient's set of signs and symptoms, history and review of systems, and point-of-care testing. Only then can intelligent treatment prioritization begin.

REFERENCES

1. Behrens A, Doyle JJ, et al. Dysfunctional tear syndrome: a Delphi approach to treatment recommendations. *Cornea.* 2006;25:8:900-7.
2. Dry Eye Workshop Panel. 2007 Report of the dry eye workshop. *Ocul Surf.* 2007;5:2:65-204.
3. Management and therapy of dry eye disease: report of the management and therapy subcommittee of the international dry eye workshop (2007). *Ocul Surf.* 2007; 5(2):163-178.
4. Bron AJ, de Paiva CS, Chauhan SK, et al. TFOS DEWS II pathophysiology report. *Ocul Surf.* 2017;15(3):438-510.
5. Blackie CA, Solomon JD, Greiner JV, Holmes M, Korb DR. Inner eyelid surface temperature as a function of warm compress methodology. *Optom Vis Sci.* 2008;85:675-683.
6. Donnenfeld ED, Mah FS, McDonald MB, et al. New considerations in the treatment of anterior and posterior blepharitis. *Refractive Eyecare.* 2008;12:3-14.

7. Pflugfelder SC, Maskin SL, Anderson B, et al. A randomized, doublemasked, placebo-controlled, multicenter comparison of loteprednol etabonate ophthalmic suspension, 0.5%, and placebo for treatment of keratoconjunctivitis sicca in patients with delayed tear clearance. *Am J Ophthalmol.* 2004;138:444-57.

8. Sall K, Stevenson OD, Mundorf TK, et al. Two multicenter, randomized studies of the efficacy and safety of cyclosporine ophthalmic emulsion in moderate to severe dry eye disease. CsA Phase 3 Study Group. *Ophthalmology.* 2000;107(4):631-639.

9. Sheppard JD, Donnenfeld, ED, Holland EJ, et. Al. Effect of loteprednol etabonate 0.5% on initiation of dry eye treatment with topical cyclosporine 0.05%. *Eye Contact Lens.* 2014;40(5):289-296.

10. Perez, VL, Pflugfelder SC, Zhang S, et al. Lifitegrast, a novel integrin antagonist for treatment of dry eye disease. *Ocul Surf.* 2016; 14: 207-215

11. Rubin M, Rao SM. Efficacy of topical cyclosporine in the treatment of posterior blepharitis. *J Ocul Pharmacol Ther.* 2006;22:47-53.

12. Foulks GN, Borchman D, Yappert M, Kim SH, McKay JW. Topical azithromycin therapy for meibomian gland dysfunction: clinical response and lipid alterations. *Cornea.* 2010;29:781-788.

13. Sheppard JD, Pflugfelder SC, et al. Long-term supplementation with n-6 and n-3 PUFAs improves moderate-to-severe keratoconjunctivitis sicca: a randomized double-blind clinical trial. *Cornea.* 2013;32:1297-1304.

14. Epitropoulos AT, Donnenfeld ED, Shah ZA, et al. Effect of oral re-esterified omega-3 nutritional supplementation on dry eyes. *Cornea.* 2016;35(9):1185-1191.

15. Balaram M, Schaumberg DA, Dana MR. Efficacy and tolerability outcomes after punctal occlusion with silicone plugs in dry eye syndrome. *Am J Ophthalmol.* 2001;131(1):30-36.

16. Brissette AR, Mednick ZD, Schweitzer KD, et. Al. Punctal plug retention rates for the treatment of moderate to severe dry eye: a randomized, double-masked, controlled clinical trial. *Am J Ophthalmol.* 2015;160(2):238-242.

17. Kashkouli MB, Fazel AJ, Kiavash V, et al. Oral azithromycin versus doxycycline in meibomian gland dysfunction: a randomised double-masked open-label clinical trial. *Br J Ophthalmol.* 2015;99(2):199-204.

18. Lane SS, DuBiner HB, Epstein RJ, et al. A new system, the LipiFlow, for the treatment of meibomian gland dysfunction. *Cornea.* 2012;31:396-404.

19. Blackie C, Carlson AN, Korb DR. Treatment for meibomian gland dysfunction and dry eye symptoms with a single-dose vectored thermal pulsation: a review. *Curr Opin Ophthalmol.* 2015;26(4):306-313.

20. He H, Li W, Tseng DY, et al. Biochemical characterization and function of complexes formed by hyaluronan and the heavy chains of inter-alpha-inhibitor (HC*HA) purified from extracts of human amniotic membrane. *J Biol Chem.* 2009;284(30):20136-20146.

21. He H, Zhang S, Tighe S, et al. Immobilized heavy chain-hyaluronic acid polarizes lipopolysaccharide-activated macrophages toward M2 phenotype. *J Biol Chem.* 2013;288(36):25792-25803.

22. Lemp MA, Bron AJ, Baudouin C, et al. Tear osmolarity in the diagnosis and management of dry eye disease. *Am J Ophthalmol.* 2011;151(5):792-798.

23. Sullivan BD, Crews LA, Sönmez B, et al. Clinical utility of objective tests for dry eye disease: variability over time and implications for clinical trials and disease management. *Cornea.* 2012;31(9): 1000-1008.

24. Cömez AT, Tufan HA, Kocabıyık O, Gencer B. Effects of lubricating agents with different osmolalities on tear osmolarity and other tear function tests in patients with dry eye. *Curr Eye Res.* 2013;38(11):1095-1103.

25. De Paiva CS, Corrales RM, Villarreal AL, et al. Corticosteroid and doxycycline suppress MMP-9 and inflammatory cytokine expression, MAPK activation in the corneal epithelium in experimental dry eye. *Exp Eye Res.* 2006;83(3):526-535.

26. Gürdal C, Genç I, Saraç O, et al. Topical cyclosporine in thyroid orbitopathy-related dry eye: clinical findings, conjunctival epithelial apoptosis, and mmp-9 expression. *Curr Eye Res.* 2010;35(9):771-777.

PART 3

Elizabeth Viriya, MD

KEY POINTS

♦ DED is multifactorial in etiology and the recommended regimen for treatment varies according to the subtype and severity.

♦ The objective of this chapter is to provide an overview of treatment in a general private practice patient population using therapeutics available in the United States.

♦ Common causes of DED include: blepharitis (MGD), aqueous deficiency, mucin deficiency, and exposure.

The ocular surface is exposed to desiccating conditions that can lead to visual disturbances, ocular discomfort, or no symptoms. In this chapter, pathology of adnexal structures that supply or maintain components of the tear film will be described. Targeted management of the underlying condition is aimed accordingly to restore homeostasis of the ocular surface, improve symptoms, resolve tissue disruption and inflammation, and prevent recurrence.

The protective liquid coating of our ocular surface ideally consists of a normoosmolar solution produced by the main and accessory lacrimal glands. The aqueous component is thickened and adherent to the ocular surface epithelium with mucins. Mucins are secreted by goblet cells, apical cells of the cornea and conjunctiva.[1] The tear film is also maintained by a lipid overlay, which prevents aqueous evaporation. These lipids, namely meibum, are secreted by the meibomian glands.

Conditions altering any component of the tear film are typically multifactorial. Causes of DED, also referred to as DTS, can be categorized functionally as: 1) blepharitis (MGD), 2) aqueous deficiency, 3) mucin deficiency, and 4) exposure (Table 15-1).[2]

OVERLAP IN TREATMENT

The targeted approach to any cause of DTS is an essential part of management. To simplify and clarify the therapeutic approach, it is worth noting the overlap in therapy. The first step is a lubricating substitute for the tear film, and when applicable, the use of anti-inflammatory medication.

Lubrication

Benefits of lubrication include improvement in symptoms, decrease in ocular surface staining, increase in TBUT, and improved Schirmer scores.[3] To avoid toxicity from preservatives in multidose formulations, preservative-free products are recommended if application exceeds 4 times a day.

The mechanisms for improvement using lubrication are unclear and perhaps due to dilution and reduction in tear hyperosmolarity, greater clearance of proinflammatory mediators and/or debris, and reduction of friction on the ocular surface.[4]

Anti-Inflammatory Agents

Tear dysfunction results in hyperosmolarity and shear stress, both of which elicit innate and autoimmune immunity[5] Inflammation exacerbates symptoms, degrades the epithelial lining, induces apoptosis of goblet cells, loss of epithelial cells, and infiltration of the lacrimal gland and ocular surface lining.[6] The consequence of inflammation is further decompensation of the ocular surface and reduction in tear production. To effectively treat DTS, the cycle of tear dysfunction and inflammation can be disrupted using the following anti-inflammatory agents.

Omega-3 Fatty Acid Supplementation

The DREAM (Dry Eye Assessment and Management) trail was a prospective, randomized, placebo-controlled study to determine efficacy of omega-3 supplementation (2 gm eicosapentaenoic acid and 1 gm docosahexaenoic acid) on signs and symptoms of moderate to severe dry eye. Both treatment and placebo led to improvement in only OSDI scores, and there was no statistically significant difference at time points 3, 6, 9, and 12 months.[7] Smaller studies have demonstrated benefits of omega-3 supplementation for dry eye and rheumatoid arthritis.[8] Given its safety of use, a trial of omega-3 supplementation can still be considered.

Steroids

Steroids are used 1 to 4 drops a day for 2 to 4 weeks for exacerbations of DTS. Corticosteroids can: 1) improve symptoms, 2) increase Schirmer scores, 3) prolong TBUT, 4) increase goblet cell density, 5) reduce ocular surface staining scores, 6) reduce conjunctival hyperemia, 7) improve marginal keratitis or phlyctenules, and 8) reduce corneal scarring.

The 2 forms of steroids are ester and ketone steroids. Ketone steroids include prednisolone, difluprednate, dexamethasone, fluorometholone, and rimexolone. The ester steroid such as loteprednol is more quickly metabolized, which lowers the risk of adverse effects such as intraocular pressure (IOP) elevation, glaucoma, posterior subcapsular cataract, and infection.

If longer duration of anti-inflammatory medication is needed, steroids can be tapered off and serve as a bridge until the onset of action with either topical CsA or lifitegrast 5% is achieved. Topical nonsteroidal anti-inflammatory drugs (eg, diclofenac) are contraindicated. Not only can it worsen DTS, but it can also cause corneal melting.

Lifitegrast 5%

Lifitegrast 5% is a neutral pH, isotonic, preservative-free antagonist of receptors on epithelial cells and other antigen presenting cells to block T-cell (CD4+) activation and

Table 15-1

Identifying Subtypes

	Blepharitis	Aqueous Deficiency	
Symptoms	Worse in the morning	Worse in the evening	
Facial Signs	Eyelash dandruff associated with rosacea Flushing Rhinophyma		
Testing	TBUT <10 seconds	Schirmer I at 5 minutes <10 mm Corneal anesthesia	
Slit-Lamp Examination Findings	Eyelid margin Hyperemia, telangiectasias, keratinization, scalloping, notching, thickening Debris (scurf, cylinders, sleeves) Meibum color, thickness, expressivity Trichiasis, madarosis Tear TBUT <10 seconds Frothy secretions Cornea Marginal infiltrates Neovascularization, pannus Scarring	Tear Tear meniscus height <0.3 mm Mucus strands Conjunctiva Injection Lissamine green staining Cornea Old incisions Fluorescein staining Epithelial defects Filaments	

IDENTIFYING SUBTYPES

MUCIN DEFICIENCY	EXPOSURE
Worse in the evening	Worse in the morning/evening
	Facial palsies Mask faces Exophthalmos Cicatricial changes
TBUT < 10 seconds	Bell's phenomenon Blink rate (normally 7 to 10 per minute) Eyelid excursion during blink

Eyelids
   Symblepharon
Conjunctiva
   Fornix foreshortening
   Keratinization
   Subepithelial fibrosis
   Trichiasis
   Bitot spots
   Lissamine green staining
Cornea
   Fluorescein staining
   Pannus
	Eyelids
	   Cicatricial changes
	Conjunctiva
	   Injection
	   Lissamine green staining
	Cornea
	   Fluorescein staining
	   Thinning
	   Ulceration
	   Scars

recruitment to the ocular surface. Long-term efficacy is still being investigated. It has a good safety profile after 1 year of continued use.[9]

Cyclosporine A 0.05%

This calcineurin inhibitor has a dual action in inflammation which: 1) inhibits proliferation of differentiated T cells and 2) prevents apoptosis of cells. Onset of action can vary from 6 weeks to 4 months. Recommended use is 1 drop twice a day (up to 4 times a day in select cases) for at least 6 months. Long-term safety has been observed for 3 years. However, after 12 months, the dose can be continued, or a trial of discontinuation, or reduction to once daily can be attempted.

The following sections discuss features of each subtype and its associated targeted therapy.

BLEPHARITIS

Pathophysiology

Blepharitis is the most common cause of patients with DTS.[10] It is characterized as inflammation involving the anterior, posterior eyelid margin, or both.

Anterior blepharitis is associated with *Staphylococcus aureus*, *Staphylococcus epidermidis*, *Propionibacterium acnes*, *Demodex*, and seborrheic dermatitis. In more advanced cases, the inflammation can extend to involve the posterior portion.

Posterior blepharitis is associated with primary or secondary MGD. Altered meibum becomes progressively more turbid and thick, and epithelial metaplasia contributes to impair expressibility of lipids until terminal duct obstruction occurs.[11] Meibomian gland loss can occur in advanced stages. MGD results from causes such as: 1) dermatologic conditions (rosacea and seborrheic blepharitis), 2) cicatricial changes (atopy, erythema multiforme, ocular cicatricial pemphigoid, and trachoma), and 3) medications (hormone replacement for postmenopausal women, antihistamines, antidepressants, and retinoids).[12]

First-Line Treatment

Eyelid Hygiene Practices

Daily or twice daily warm compresses and eyelid hygiene can benefit nearly all forms of blepharitis. Warm compress with eyelid massage softens eyelid debris and promotes expressibility of abnormal, thickened meibum. Eyelid cleansing with commercially available cleansers or nonirritating shampoo reduce debris and bacterial load.

Lubrication

Formulations with more lipid content have been suggested to supplement the deficient lipid production in MGD.

Omega-3 Fatty Acid Supplementation

Studies suggest use can improve symptoms, meibum quality, and TBUT.[13]

Second-Line Treatment

Indications

Further management is indicated for blepharitis that is refractory to conservative measures and/or more advanced. For anterior blepharitis: 1) eyelid telangiectasias, hyperemia, ulcerations, 2) ocular surface staining, or 3) symptoms. For posterior blepharitis: 1) presence of symptoms, 2) meibum that is not clear, 3) inability to express meibum on manual compression from more than half of the surveyed glands (see grading system from the International Workshop on Meibomian Gland Dysfunction), or 4) ocular surface staining.[14]

Topical Antibiotic Use

Since anterior blepharitis is related to bacterial load and toxins, topical antibiotics are recommended. Bacitracin is a bactericidal agent used for overgrowth of Gram-positive pathogens such as *S. aureus* and *S. epidermidis*. Metronidazole 1% gel is indicated for rosacea associated blepharitis. Tea tree oil (20% to 50%) applied weekly or daily, or tea tree shampoo use for 6 weeks is recommended for demodicosis.[15]

Macrolides such as azithromycin and erythromycin can be used off-label for anterior and posterior blepharitis. It is bacteriostatic and also has anti-inflammatory properties (ie, reduces lipase production, inhibits recruitment of immune cells, and decreases expression of cytokines and chemokines). Clinical trials have demonstrated suggested improvement in meibomian gland expressivity, secretion clarity, TBUT, and ocular surface staining with topical azithromycin. Similar improvement can be achieved with oral administration, but caution is advised given the risk of serious heart arrhythmias and gastrointestinal (GI) side effects.

Systemic Antibiotic/Anti-Inflammatory Medication

In cases of MGD, a trial of systemic antibiotics with anti-inflammatory properties are recommended. Tetracyclines and their derivatives, namely doxycycline or minocycline, impair neutrophil recruitment, and activation of lymphocytes, decrease lipase and MMP-9 production independent of its bacteriostatic effects. Nursing or pregnant women and children should avoid use. Adverse effects include photosensitization, GI upset, vaginitis, azotemia, and pseudotumor cerebri. Tetracycline can also reduce the efficacy of warfarin and oral contraceptives.

Third-Line Treatment

Indications

Adjunctive anti-inflammatory agents can benefit patients when blepharitis presents with: 1) moderate or marked symptoms, 2) ocular surface staining grade > 23 by NEI/

Industry grading system or > 10 by the Oxford scale, 3) any central staining or corneal neovascularization, or 4) conjunctival hyperemia/phlectenules.[16]

Topical Anti-Inflammatory

Anti-inflammatory agents including steroids, lifitegrast 5%, or CsA are mainly for exacerbations of inflammation from tear instability and associated aqueous tear deficiency. However, studies suggest CsA can decrease eyelid margin hyperemia, telangiectasia, and corneal staining.[17]

Systemic Management

In the setting of dermatologic or systemic conditions that contribute to blepharitis, referral for comanagement with a primary doctor, rheumatologist, or dermatologist can also be considered. For example, severe rosacea or androgen deficiency.

For a summary of management for anterior vs posterior blepharitis, see Table 15-2 and 15-3.

AQUEOUS TEAR DEFICIENCY

Pathophysiology

This category encompasses a group of disorders affecting aqueous tear supply. Deficiency can result from any or a combination of the following: 1) neurotrophic ocular surface, 2) reduced innervation to the lacrimal glands, 3) primary or secondary Sjögren syndrome or age-related infiltration of fibrosis of lacrimal glands that produce the aqueous component of tears, and 4) inflammatory or cicatricial changes that impede or obstruct flow through lacrimal ducts onto the ocular surface.

First-Line Therapy

Avoiding Exogenous Factors

A person's environmental or personal risk factors can help reduce symptoms and severity of dry eye. For example: 1) avoiding heat, air currents, low humidity, or wearing moisture chamber eyewear/shields, 2) voluntary eye closure intermittently during prolonged upward gaze or visually demanding tasks, 3) limiting instillation of topical medications, especially if it contains benzalkonium chloride (BAK), which can cause epithelial toxicity, 4) avoiding systemic medications that can reduce tear secretion, such as systemic antihistamines and psychiatric medications with anticholinergic effects, 5) eyelid margin hygiene to reduce concomitant blepharitis, or 6) avoiding smoking.

Lubrication

An additional modality of lubricating the ocular surface can be done by placing a hydroxypropyl cellulose insert, Lacrisert (Aton Pharmaceuticals), in the inferior

TABLE 15-2

SUMMARY OF ANTERIOR BLEPHARITIS TREATMENT	
ANTERIOR BLEPHARITIS	**MANAGEMENT**
Asymptomatic No ocular surface staining Eyelid debris	Warm compress ≥4 minutes 1 to 2 times a day Eyelid scrubs with moderate to firm massage Artificial tears 4 times a day; as needed

Symptomatic
Eyelid Margin
  Hyperemia
  Telangiectasia
  Ulcers
  Ocular surface staining
	All the above, plus omega-3 supplementation and any one of the following:
	  Bacitracin ophthalmic ointment every day at bedtime or twice a day.
	  Erythromycin ophthalmic ointment twice a day or every day at bedtime
	  Azithromycin 1 drop twice a day for 2 days then every day for 2 to 4 weeks.

Phylectenules Marginal Infiltrates Corneal Neovascularization/ Scarring	All the above, plus: Steroids 1 to 4 times a day for 2 to 4 weeks

cul-de-sac that slowly dissolves to increase tear film viscosity. If used, insertion once daily is sufficient, or twice if placed additionally in the evening.

Omega-3 Fatty Acid Supplementation

Studies suggest improvement in symptoms, TBUT, osmolarity, and conjunctival injection.[18]

Topical Anti-Inflammatory

Therapeutic options include steroids, lifitegrast 5%, or CsA. CsA demonstrated statistically significant improvement in ocular surface staining, 59% improved Schirmer scores, better vision, and decreased need for lubrication.[19] Lifitegrast 5% applied twice a day can improve symptoms and signs of dry eye as early as 2 weeks. Studies have shown improvement in symptoms and staining scores.[20]

TABLE 15-3

SUMMARY OF POSTERIOR BLEPHARITIS TREATMENT

POSTERIOR BLEPHARITIS/ MEIBOMIAN GLAND DYSFUNCTION	MANAGEMENT
Asymptomatic No ocular surface staining >50% glands expressible Minimally altered meibum	Warm compress ≥4 minutes once or twice a day Eyelid scrubs with moderate to firm massage Artificial tears 4 times a day; as needed

Symptoms of ocular discomfort, itchiness, photophobia, burning in the morning, and any of the following:
  Clear to cloudy meibum
  Expressibility of >50% meibomian glands
  Ocular surface staining:
    Occassional
	All the above, plus omega-3 supplementation and any one of the following:
	  Erythromycin ophthalmic ointment every day at bedtime or twice a day
	  Azithromycin 1 drop twice a day for 2 days then every day for 12 to 26 days

Some limitations of activities because of symptoms and any of the following:
  Eyelid margin telangiectasias
  Diffuse meibum clouding, granularity, thickening
  <50% gland expressibility
  Peripheral corneal staining
	Switch topical antibiotics to:
	  Doxycycline or minocycline 50 to 100 mg by mouth, every day or twice a day for 2 to 6 weeks (especially if there is concomitant rosacea)
	  Then taper

Disability from symptoms and:
  Granular and thick meibum
  Poor expressibility—extensive gland dropout
  Central corneal staining
  Conjunctival hyperemia and staining
	All the above and an anti-inflammatory
	  Steroids (FML, Lotemax) every day to 4 times a day for 2 to 4 weeks
	  And consider:
	    Restasis 1 drop twice a day
	    Lifitegrast 5% 1 drop twice a day

Second-Line Therapy

Oral Secretagogues

Oral secretagogues stimulate lacrimal and salivary gland secretion. Pilocarpine and cevimeline are FDA-approved for oral symptoms caused by Sjögren syndrome, and use for dry eye is off-label. Approximately 40% of patients on either secretagogue feel improvement in ocular symptoms. Pilocarpine has been shown to reduce rose bengal staining and increasing goblet cell density.[21] Adverse effects may include sweating, urinary frequency, flushing, and chills. Cevimeline use is generally better tolerated than pilocarpine. Referral to a rheumatologist or a primary care physician to direct dosing and titration is recommended.

Tear Retention

Punctal occlusion/stenosis retain lacrimal secretions to reduce symptoms, ocular surface staining, and improve tear stability and Schirmer scores. Some evidence recommends treating surface inflammation prior to plug insertion. A trial with dissolvable plugs might be trialed to rule out iatrogenic epiphora. At 2 years after implantation, about half will have extruded spontaneously. Caution must be exercised to prevent internal migration which may result in nasolacrimal duct obstruction.

Autologous Serum

Autologous serum and other blood products provide lubrication as well as Vitamin A, cytokines, epidermal growth factor, neurotrophic growth factor, and anti-inflammatory substances, such as interleukin receptor antagonists and inhibitors of MMP-9.[22] Serum can improve symptoms, fluorescein TBUT, and rose bengal staining scores. Concentrations of 20% to 100% can be applied 4 to 8 times a day and titrated according to clinical response. Proper storage instructions are important to follow because all preparations are preservative free. Used vials require refrigeration and unused vials must be kept frozen.

Therapeutic Contact Lenses

Therapeutic or bandage soft contact lenses can promote corneal healing in cases of severe corneal staining, epithelial defects, or filamentary keratitis. It shields the ocular surface from the eyelids and environment, reduces desiccation, improves vision, and relieves pain. Contact lenses suitable for use as a bandage must have high oxygen diffusion (D/k). Recommended brands include: Air Optix Night and Day Aqua (Alcon), PureVision (Bausch + Lomb), Acuvue Oasys (Vistakon), and Sof-Form 55EW (Unilens). If use of the contact lens extends beyond a few days, consider adding prophylactic antibiotic. Close monitoring is advised to avoid infectious keratitis, corneal edema, or melting.

Rigid scleral contact lenses or Prosthetic Replacement of the Ocular Surface Ecosystem (PROSE) is a gas permeable material that vaults over the cornea with an aqueous reservoir, which lubricates and protects the ocular surface. The added advantage is significant improvement in vision even with highly aberrant corneas. Scleral contact lenses for routine use should be removed before sleeping. However, if corneal healing is the objective, extended wear with prophylactic antibiotics can be considered.

Amniotic Membrane Bandage

Amniotic membrane transplantation (AMT) can be utilized as an anti-inflammatory bandage for several days. Its mechanism of action includes: 1) entrapment and apoptosis of immune cells, 2) barrier against microtrauma and desiccation, and 3) source of growth factors that either directly or indirectly improve corneal sensation.[23] AMT use can obscure vision and can be performed by using a self-contained ring such as PROKERA (Bio-Tissue) and tape tarsorrhaphy to prevent prolapse of the device. Or, the AM can be held in place with a soft contact lens overlay for a few days.

Systemic Management

The incidence of Sjögren syndrome is reportedly 10% of the dry eye population.[24,25] Association with dry mouth, arthralgias, myalgias, and malaise should warrant suspicion. The ocular surface can improve with systemic management of Sjögren syndrome and collagen vascular diseases. Comanaging with a rheumatologist may be considered, especially if there is a lack of familiarity with systemic anti-inflammatory medications.

For a summary of management for aqueous tear deficiency, see Table 15-4.

MUCIN DEFICIENCY

Pathophysiology

Mucin production is dependent on the density of secretory cells and parasympathetic innervation. Mucin deficiency causes tear instability and reduces TBUT. The etiology results from inflammation, cicatricial conjunctival conditions, and Vitamin A deficiency. Similar to aqueous tear deficiency, the recommendations are tailored to the cause.

First-Line Therapy

Avoid Offending Agents

Pseudopemphigoid can improve with discontinuation of offending agents, such as echothiophate iodide, epinephrine, pilocarpine, or timolol eyedrops.

Xerophthalmia

Deficient Vitamin A serum level can be supplemented with high oral doses. Close monitoring is required because of potential toxicity from indiscriminate Vitamin A intake.

Autoimmune Cicatricial Disorders

Autoimmune conditions, such as ocular cicatricial pemphigoid, can be suppressed by systemic steroids as well as other systemic immunomodulatory agents ("steroid-sparing" agents). Management with a rheumatologist is highly recommended.

TABLE 15-4

SUMMARY OF AQUEOUS TEAR DEFICIENCY MANAGEMENT	
PRESENTATION	**TREATMENT**
Symptoms (burning, foreign body sensation, intermittent blurring) Little to no ocular surface changes Tear meniscus < 0.3 mm Schirmer or Schirmer I < 10 mm at 5 minutes	Avoiding environmental or situational triggers Lubrication Consider omega-3 fatty acid supplementation

Moderate to severe ocular staining
Conjunctival hyperemia
Filaments
	All the above and steroid (every day to 4 times a say for 2 to 4 weeks).
	And consider:
	    Restasis 1 drop twice a day for 6 to 12 months, or
	    Lifitegrast 5% 1 drop twice a day for 6 to 12 months

Diffuse epithelial staining
Epithelial defects
Scarring
	All the above and any or a combination of the following options:
	    Secretagogues
	        Pilocarpine 5 mg 4 times a day
	        Cevimeline 30 mg 3 times a day
	    Autologous serum 20% to 100%, 4 to 8 times a day
	    Therapeutic contact lens
	    Amniotic membrane placement
	    Punctal occlusion

Lubrication

Tear substitutes provide symptomatic relief and reduce further frictional forces on epitheliopathy with repetitive blinks.

Topical Anti-Inflammatory

These agents include omega-3 supplementation, pulsed topical steroids, CsA, or lifitegrast 5%. FDA studies on CsA shows that goblet cell density increased by as much a 191%.

Second-Line Therapy

Eye Cover/Protection

In cases where there is an irreversible loss or severe mucin deficiency, then moisture chamber eyewear or scleral contact lenses may be indicated.

EXPOSURE

Pathophysiology

Impaired eyelid closure with prolonged desiccation of the ocular surface can cause ocular surface breakdown and symptoms. The differential includes: 1) impaired blinking whether from CN VII palsy, Parkinson's disease, supranuclear palsy, visually intent tasks, or anesthetic abuse, 2) obstruction to blink such as ocular surface masses, exophthalmos, or shallow orbits, or 3) eyelid malposition such as lagophthalmos and ectropion.

The patient's Bell's phenomenon should be assessed to determine the extent of ocular surface protection required.

First-Line Therapy

Blink Exercises

Blinking normally occurs 7 to 10 times a minute. This motion effectively clears away debris, rinses fresh tears over the surface, and compresses the meibomian glands to express meibum. There is no consensus on the type of exercise that will produce muscle memory to consistently improve eyelid closure, but a sequence of repetitive eyelid squeezing multiple times a day has been suggested.

Lubrication

As with other subtypes of DTS mentioned above, lubrication, or tear retention using a moisture chamber is indicated.

Correcting Eyelid Position

To reduce the exposed surface area, eyelid taping can serve as a temporizing measure. Referral to oculoplastics is recommended for definitive management.

Topical Anti-Inflammatory

May include a short course of steroids, and/or CsA or lifitegrast 5% for long-term control of inflammation.

Amniotic Membrane

Described in further detail in the aqueous tear deficiency section, AM facilitates healing, especially for epithelial breakdown or corneal thinning.

Second-Line Therapy

Scleral Contact Lenes

Scleral contact lenses may provide relief and protection, but cautious monitoring is required. Prophylactic antibiotic use can be considered if used chronically.

SUMMARY

Persistent risk factors that desiccate the ocular surface require long-term management to prevent recurrent episodes. The multifactorial process can be tempered with a targeted approach based on the tear film constituent that is altered. To date, there is no standardized algorithm. The busy practicing clinician is best suited to determine the optimal regimen on a case-by-case basis. The compilation of guidelines from the International Workshop on Meibomian Gland Dysfunction, DEWS, and DEWS II can help guide current therapy given the current understanding of the DTS.

REFERENCES

1. Ablamowicz AF, Nichols JJ. Ocular Surface Membrane-Associated Mucins. *Ocul Surf.* 2016;14(3):331-341.
2. Milner MS, Beckman KA, Luchs JI, et al. Dysfunctional tear syndrome: dry eye disease and associated tear film disorders new strategies for diagnosis and treatment. *Curr Opin Ophthalmol.* 2017;28:3-47.
3. Management and therapy of dry eye disease: report of the management and therapy subcommittee of the international dry eye workshop (2007). *Ocul Surf.* 2007;5(2):163-178.
4. Moshirfar M, Pierson K, Hanamaikai K, Santiago-Caban L, Muthappan V, Passi SF. Artificial tears potpourri: a literature review. *Clin Ophthalmol.* 2014;8:1419-1433.
5. The definition and classification of dry eye disease: report of the definition and classification subcommittee of the international dry eye workshop (2007). *Ocul Surf.* 2007;5:75-92.
6. Perez VL, Pflugfelder SC, Zhang S, Shojaei A, Haque R. Lifitegrast, a novel integrin antagonist for treatment of dry eye disease. *Ocul Surf.* 2016;14:207-215.
7. Wei Y, Asbell P. The core mechanism of dry eye disease is inflammation. *Eye Contact Lens.* 2014;40:248-256.
8. Dry Eye Assessment and Management Study Research Group, Asbell PA, Maguire MG, et al. n-3 fatty acid supplementation for the treatment of dry eye disease. *N Engl J Med.* 2018;378(18):1681-1690.
9. Donnenfeld E, Karpecki PM, Majmudar PA, et al. Safety of lifitegrast ophthalmic solution 5.0% in patients with dry eye disease: a 1-year, multicenter, randomized, placebo-controlled study. *Cornea.* 2016;35:741-748.
10. Nichols KN, Foulks GN, Bron AJ, et al. The international workshop on meibomian gland Dysfunction: executive summary. *Invest Ophthalmol Vis Sci.* 2011;52:922-1929.
11. Tomlinson A, Bron AJ, Korb DR, et al. The international workshop on meibomian gland dysfunction: report of the diagnosis subcommittee. *Invest Ophthalmol Vis Sci.* 2011;52(4):2006-2049.

12. Schaumberg DA, Nichols JJ, Papas EB, Tong L, Uchino M, Nichols KK. The international workshop on meibomian gland dysfunction: report of the subcommittee on the epidemiology of, and associated risk factors for, MGD. *Invest Ophthalmol Vis Sci.* 2011;52(4):1994-2005.

13. Macsai, MS. The role of omega-3 dietary supplementation in blepharitis and meibomian gland dysfunction (an AOS thesis). *Trans Am Ophthalmol Soc.* 2008;106:336-356.

14. Geerling G, Tauber J, Baudouin C, et al. The international workshop on meibomian gland dysfunction: report of the subcommittee on management and treatment of meibomian gland dysfunction. *Invest Ophthalmol Vis Sci.* 2011;52(4):2050-2064

15. American Academy of Ophthalmology. Blepharitis Preferred Practice Pattern. American Academy of Ophthalmology Web site. https://www.aaojournal.org/article/S0161-6420(18)32645-9/pdf. Updated October, 2018.

16. Bron A, Evans VE, Smith JA. Grading of corneal and conjunctival staining in the context of other dry eye tests. *Cornea.* 2003;22(7):640-650.

17. Perry HD, Doshi-Carnevale S, Donnenfeld ED, Solomon R, Biser SA, Bloom AH. Efficacy of commercially available topical cyclosporin A 0.05% in the treatment of meibomian gland dysfunction. *Cornea.* 2006;25:171-175.

18. Deinema LA, Vingrys AJ, Wong CY, Jackson DC, Chinnery HR, Downie LE. A randomized, double-masked, placebo-controlled clinical trial of two forms of omega-3 supplements for treating dry eye disease. *Ophthalmology.* 2017;124(1):43-52.

19. Stevenson W, Chauhan SK, Dana R. Dry eye disease: an immune-mediated ocular surface disorder. *Arch Ophthalmol.* 2012;130:90-100.

20. Semba C, Gadek T. Development of lifitegrast: a novel T-cell inhibitor for the treatment of dry eye disease. *Clin Ophthalmol.* 2016;10:1083-1094.

21. Foulks GN, Forstot SL, Donshik PC, et al. Clinical guidelines for management of dry eye associated with sjögren disease. *Ocul Surf.* 2015;13(2):118-132.

22. Ambroziak A, , Szaflik J, Szaflik JP, Ambroziak M, Witkiewicz J, Skopiński P. Immunomodulation on the ocular surface: a review. *Cent Eur J Immunol.* 2016;41:195-208.

23. Cheng AM, Zhao D, Chen R, et al. Accelerated restoration of ocular surface health in dry eye disease by self-retained cryopreserved amniotic membrane. *Ocul Surf.* 2016;14:56-63.

24. Akpek EK, Klimava A, Thorne JE, et al. Evaluation of patients with dry eye for presence of underlying Sjogren syndrome. *Cornea* 2009;28(5):493-497.

25. Liew MS, Zhang M, Kim E, Akpek EK. Prevalence and predictors of Sjogren's syndrome in a prospective cohort of patients with aqueous-deficient dry eye. *Br J Ophthalmol.* 2012;96(12):1498-1503.

SECTION IV

DEVICES AND PROCEDURES FOR DRY EYE

CHAPTER 16

Advances in Therapeutic Contact Lenses

Bandage Contact Lenses, Prosthetic Replacement of the Ocular Surface Ecosystem Treatment

Christos Theophanous, MD and Deborah S. Jacobs, MD

KEY POINTS

◆ Both soft and large diameter rigid gas permeable contact lenses can serve as a therapeutic option after trauma or surgery, and in the management of ocular surface disease.

◆ Contact lens wear is a risk factor for microbial keratitis. There are no standard guidelines as to the use of prophylactic antibiotics during therapeutic contact lens wear. Considerations include if the patient is postoperative or has a frank epithelial defect since medicamentosa and emergence of resistant microbes may occur with long-term use.

◆ Therapeutic contact lenses have been used in ocular chronic graft-versus-host disease, Sjögren syndrome, and persistent epithelial defects.

◆ Prosthetic Replacement of the Ocular Surface Ecosystem (PROSE) treatment plays a role in the management of ocular surface disease that has failed standard therapy such as bandage soft contact lenses.

Mah FS, Rhee MK, eds.
Dry Eye Disease: A Practical Guide (pp 189-197).
© 2019 Taylor & Francis Group.

Contact lenses are more than a cosmetic alternative to glasses. Contact lenses can serve as a therapeutic option after trauma or surgery and in the management of ocular surface disease. Both soft contact lenses and large diameter rigid gas permeable contact lenses can serve in these roles.

There are contact lenses that are labelled by the US Food and Drug Administration (FDA) with therapeutic indications for use (IFU), including certain Silicone-Hydrogel (Si-Hy) soft contact lenses, certain methafilcon hydrogel contact lenses, and the scleral contact lens prosthetic devices used in Prosthetic Replacement of the Ocular Surface Ecosystem (PROSE) treatment. Contact lenses with therapeutic IFU are generally characterized by high gas permeability to allow oxygen delivery to the healing or diseased ocular surface. It is also not uncommon for physicians to use contact lenses labelled only for the correction of refractive error in healthy eyes on an off-label basis for therapeutic purposes.

Contact lens use can be associated with complications such as neovascularization and microbial keratitis. With informed choices regarding contact lens design, material, and mode of wear, clinicians can reduce the likelihood of such complications in patients already at risk.

HISTORY: THE BANDAGE CONTACT LENS

Contact, as opposed to spectacle lenses, were developed in the late 19th century in Europe.[1] They were made of blown glass and used for the correction of very high refractive errors. Contact lenses have traditionally served a cosmetic purpose, providing an alternative to spectacles for correction of refractive error. With the introduction of plastics (Poly[methyl methacrylate]) to the field, "hard" contact lenses could be made smaller and lighter leading to widespread use. However, even through the 1970s, a critical deficiency persisted: contact lenses were largely impermeable to oxygen. Large contact lenses put patients at high risk for corneal edema, opacification, and neovascularization, and small contact lenses required adaptation for tolerance and were suitable for use only in eyes with healthy ocular surfaces.

Significant breakthroughs occurred in the 1970s with the introduction of "soft" hydrogel contact lenses, whose higher water content allowed for the transmission of oxygen. Gas permeable plastics were also introduced for use in "hard" contact lenses making them rigid gas permeable.

These improvements in contact lens materials laid the foundation for therapeutic application of contact lenses. Manufacturers began marketing contact lenses specifically for therapeutic usage and bandage contact lenses were brought to market for the protection of the ocular surface after trauma, to promote wound healing, and to relieve pain. The Plano T (Bausch + Lomb) was an early bandage contact lens that was used to promote epithelialization and seal leaks. The Permalens (CooperVision), a thicker and higher power contact lens, was approved for therapeutic correction of aphakia to be worn on extended wear (EW) basis with monthly replacement.

Bandage contact lenses were further utilized to provide pain relief. They found application for painful episodes in patients with aphakic and pseudophakic bullous keratopathy (BK). With the advent of laser refractive surgery, surgeons and their patients quickly appreciated the role of hydrogel soft contact lenses for postoperative symptom relief and promotion of healing after excimer laser surface ablation. Gas permeable plastics, modern lathe techniques, and computer aided design and manufacture (CAD/CAM) allowed for the design of scleral contact lenses, such as those used in PROSE treatment, that could also serve as a bandage.

Today, therapeutic contact lenses are used for dry eye disease (DED) including a variety of ocular surface disorders, after trauma, and routinely following surface ablation and epithelium off cross-linking. Bandage soft contact lenses are more commonly utilized for short-term indications while PROSE treatment is more appropriate for longer-term use.

REGULATORY MATTERS

Contact lenses are considered medical devices. In the United States, the FDA plays an important role in assuring that all medical devices, including contact lenses, are safe and effective as marketed. Approval and labelling are specific to IFU and mode of wear. For instance, approval for EW, which is a mode of wear, does not mean a contact lens is approved for therapeutic use, and vice versa. A marketed contact lens is also characterized by material (with features such as water content and gas permeability), design (shape of the contact lens including a range of diameters), and optical features. Contact lenses are marketed with an IFU related to the correction of refractive error in healthy eyes. There are a few contact lenses with therapeutic IFU typically listed as corneal protection, corneal pain relief, and use as a bandage/barrier during the healing process, but not labeled for specific diseases. It is not uncommon for physicians to use contact lenses labelled only for the correction of refraction error in healthy eyes on an off-label basis for therapeutic purposes.

As mentioned above, mode of wear or use is independent of IFU. A particular contact lens is labelled for EW (use under closed eyelids) as opposed to planned replacement daily wear (less than 24 hours then cleaned, disinfected, and reused for a specified interval of time) or as daily disposable (DD—used less than 24 hours and then discarded). The scleral contact lens prosthetic device used in PROSE treatment is labeled for therapeutic use. These devices are individually customized, large diameter, rigid gas permeable contact lenses that rest on the conjunctiva over the sclera, vaulting the cornea, allowing for the physiologic function of a diseased ocular surface. The reservoir is filled with sterile saline at the time of application onto the surface of the eye. The device is worn on a DW basis with removal before sleep for cleaning and overnight disinfection. The devices used in PROSE treatment are labelled for therapeutic purposes for distorted corneas and certain disorders of the ocular surface. It is not uncommon for physicians to use other scleral contact lenses which are labelled for irregular cornea in healthy eyes for therapeutic purposes.[2,3]

There is no soft contact lens labeled specifically for dry eye. However, the Proclear (CooperVision) series of contact lenses carries an FDA label stating that it "may provide improved comfort for contact lens wearers who experience mild discomfort or symptoms relating to dryness during contact lens wear."[4] Among soft contact lenses, a misconception is that higher water contact lenses will reduce dry eye symptoms in contact lens wearers. Clinical experience is that the highest water content hydrogels may act as sponges and be adherent rather than physiologic in dry eye. Tear exchange, contact lens fit, edge design, and lubricity are just a few of the factors other than water content that play a role in contact lens comfort. Measures worth considering for patients with contact lens intolerance related to dry eye include punctal occlusion, change of care system from multipurpose solution to peroxide system, or elimination of care system by switching to a DD contact lens. The contact lens industry has introduced innovations such as gradient contact lenses, material modifications, and surface modification to improve comfort in soft contact lenses, but it is worth noting that dry eye is not specifically an IFU for any soft contact lens.[5]

CONTACT LENS SELECTION

When soft contact lenses are used on a therapeutic basis after trauma or surgery, they are typically worn on an EW basis for a short period of time. Si-Hy contact lenses introduced over a decade ago are among the few contact lenses that do carry therapeutic labeling and EW labeling, and for those reasons are a good choice. These contact lenses sought to improve on hydrogel contact lenses by introducing a silicone polymer that would increase oxygen permeability. When initially developed, these contact lenses were expected to reduce the risk of infection compared to conventional hydrogels when worn on the same EW basis. Early reports were favorable regarding the therapeutic application of Si-Hy contact lenses for a variety of conditions.[6] Epidemiologic data has revealed little to no reduction in infection rates compared to hydrogel contact lenses with EW in general use,[6,7] suggesting that hypoxia is only one variable in the development of infection.

There are 3 Si-Hy contact lenses labelled for EW and with therapeutic IFU (Table 16-1), making them good choices as a therapeutic contact lens. Contact lenses intended for DD, although less expensive, are not designed or approved for EW and are not good options for therapeutic use.

The Kontur contact lens (Kontur Kontact Lens) is a large diameter hydrogel lens that is a good choice when the more standard diameter (approximately 14 mm) Si-Hy contact lenses are poorly retained. The Kontur contact lens is not labelled for therapeutic use, although other contact lenses made of the same material carry therapeutic labelling (see Table 16-1). The Kontur contact lens is generally well tolerated in diameters of 16 mm, 18 mm, and larger, and is the default choice for maintenance of hydration over Boston Keratoprosthesis.[9,10] The larger diameters are available with independent choice of base curve for the central optic zone and base curve for the peripheral outer zone, to allow for better alignment and retention in the larger diameters. Of note, the Kontur contact lens is of low oxygen permeability and is not a good choice for corneas in which neovascularization is to be avoided.

Contact lens intended for EW, especially in an eye made vulnerable by trauma, surgery, or disease, should be undertaken with caution since overnight wear increases the risk of infection and hypoxic insult. Duration of EW should be limited to the shortest

TABLE 16-1

CONTACT LENSES LABELLED WITH THERAPEUTIC INDICATION FOR USE

MANUFACTURER	TRADE NAME	LENS MATERIAL	USAGE DURATION	TRANSMISSIBILITY (DK)	WATER CONTENT (%)
Vistakon	Acuvue Oasys	Senofilcon A	7 days	147	38
Bausch + Lomb	PureVision2	Balafilcon A	30 days	130	36
Alcon	Air Optix Night & Day Aqua	Lotrafilcon A	30 days	175	24
Unilens	Sof-Form 55 EW	Methfilcon A	7 days	18.8	55
United Contact Lens	UCL 55/46	Ocufilcon C/A	7 days	18.8/15/25	55/46
BostonSight	BostonSightPD	Equalens II	Daily Wear	85	N/A
		XO2		141	
		Optimum Extra		100	
		Optimum Extreme		125	

period possible. Soft contact lenses should be replaced or cleaned by the clinician at appropriate intervals. For patients who require long-term therapeutic contact lenses for chronic ocular surface disease, training in insertion, removal, and contact lens disinfec tion by the patient or caregiver should be undertaken with the goal of routine cleaning or replacement at home and eventually conversion to daily wear.

COMPLICATIONS AND RISK FACTORS

Contact lens wear is a risk factor for microbial keratitis. Pathogens can be introduced through a variety of mechanisms—from the wearer's finger during insertion, the eyelid margin, the storage case, or contact lens solution.[11] Lack of epithelial integrity and con-comitant use of topical or systemic steroids also increase infection risk.

There are no standard guidelines as to the use of prophylactic antibiotics during therapeutic contact lens wear. In an older study of BK, risk factors for infection were duration of BK, steroid use, and bandage contact lens use. Use of topical antibiotics was not protective.[12] Common choices for prophylaxis are fluoroquinolones, polymyxin/trimethoprim, or aminoglycosides used twice a day to 4 times a day. Antibiotics which have low toxicity profiles or are preservative free should be considered for patients with underlying ocular surface disease. It is our practice to use topical antibiotic prophylaxis only in postoperative cases or when there is a geographic epithelial defect, but not for therapeutic contact lens wear over punctate keratitis—the rationale being that long-term use can lead to medicamentosa and to emergence of resistant microbial organisms.

Corneal neovascularization and opacification are potential complications of thera-peutic contact lens usage. In patients with underlying ocular surface disease, it can be difficult to distinguish whether these complications represent progression of underlying disease or a response to contact lenses. Contact lenses with lower oxygen permeability or poor fit can lead to neovascularization, and in such cases, change to a different contact lens material or design may be warranted if discontinuation is not feasible.

REPORTS OF CONTACT LENSES USED IN DRY EYE DISEASE

There is a growing body of literature on the role of therapeutic contact lens in the treatment of DED.

Chronic Graft-Versus-Host Disease

Ocular chronic graft-versus-host disease (cGVHD) is particularly amenable to management with therapeutic contact lens especially as standard management of DED provides inadequate relief for a substantial fraction of patients. There are reports of sig-nificant positive impact on comfort and vision with soft contact lenses,[13,14] with scleral contact lenses,[15] and with PROSE treatment.[16-18]

Prophylactic antibiotics were used in both reports of soft contact lens use, but not with PROSE treatment except when there is a geographic epithelial defect. In that case, one drop of preservative-free moxifloxacin is added to the reservoir. Persistent symptoms and signs may be indicative of inadequate systemic therapy and coordinating management with a patient's oncologist may be required.[19]

Sjögren Syndrome

The value of bandage soft contact lenses in Sjögren syndrome patients has been demonstrated.[20] There are reports of scleral contact lens use and PROSE treatment in ocular surface disease cohorts that include Sjögren syndrome patients.[21-24] As with other applications, therapeutic contact lenses can provide ocular surface protection, promote healing, reduce desiccation, and alleviate pain for Sjögren syndrome patients.

Persistent Epithelial Defects

Protection from environmental and eyelid insult can be particularly important in treating persistent epithelial defects (PEDs). Contact lenses labeled for EW or that have high oxygen permeability are best suited for these patients. In these cases, particular care should be given to achieving optimal contact lens fit to improve patient comfort and healing. Use of prophylactic antibiotics is warranted and consideration should be given to choices and regimens that minimize toxicity and exposure to preservatives. A combination of bandage soft contact lenses with autologous serum has demonstrated benefit for PEDs.[25,26]

PROSE treatment can also promote healing of PEDs. When other treatment modalities have been unsuccessful, off-label continuous wear of PROSE devices can be considered. A high rate of microbial keratitis in an early report[27] has apparently been addressed with standard management regimens and with the introduction of non-preserved fluoroquinolone to the device chamber at the time of insertion.[28-31] PROSE treatment can succeed in the management of PEDs after the use of bandage soft contact lenses have failed.[30]

SUMMARY

There have been substantial innovations in the field of therapeutic contact lens over the past 2 decades. High oxygen transmissible soft contact lenses can be useful for the protection of the cornea, promotion of healing, and reduction of pain after trauma and surgery and in certain clinical situations. PROSE treatment plays a role in the management of ocular surface disease that has failed standard approaches including the use of bandage soft contact lenses. Therapeutic contact lenses are an important option for clinicians managing patients with dry eye and ocular surface disease.

REFERENCES

1. Fick AE. A contact lens. 1888. *Arch Ophthalmol.* 1997;115(1):120-121.
2. Schornack MM. Scleral lenses: a literature review. *Eye Contact Lens.* 2015;41(1):3-11.
3. van der Worp E, Bornman D, Ferreira DL, et al. Modern scleral contact lenses: a review. *Cont Lens Anterior Eye.* 2014;37(4):240-250.
4. CooperVision. US Food and Drug Administration Web site. https://www.accessdata.fda.gov/cdrh_docs/pdf6/K061948.pdf. Published November 22, 2006.
5. Papas EB, Ciolino JB, Jacobs D, et al. The TFOS International Workshop on Contact Lens Discomfort: report of the management and therapy subcommittee. *Invest Ophthalmol Vis Sci.* 2013;54(11):TFOS183-203.
6. Kanpolat A, Uçakhan OO. Therapeutic use of focus night & day contact lenses. *Cornea.* 2003;22(8):726-734.
7. Stapleton F, Keay L, Edwards K, et al. The incidence of contact lens-related microbial keratitis in Australia. *Ophthalmology.* 2008;115(10):1655-1662.
8. Dart JK, Radford CF, Minassian D, Verma S, Stapleton F. Risk factors for microbial keratitis with contemporary contact lenses: a case-control study. *Ophthalmology.* 2008;115(10):1647-1654.
9. Dohlman CH, Dudenhoefer EJ, Khan BF, Morneault S. Protection of the ocular surface after kerato-prosthesis surgery: the role of soft contact lenses. *CLAO J.* 2002;28(2):72-74.
10. Beyer J, Todani A, Dohlman C. Prevention of visually debilitating deposits on soft contact lenses in keratoprosthesis patients. *Cornea.* 2011;30(12):1419-1422.
11. Fleiszig SM, Evans DJ. Pathogenesis of contact lens-associated microbial keratitis. *Optom Vis Sci.* 2010;87(4):225-232.
12. Luchs JI, Cohen EJ, Rapuano CJ, Laibson PR. Ulcerative keratitis in bullous keratopathy. *Ophthalmology.* 1997;104(5):816-822.
13. Inamoto Y, Sun YC, Flowers ME, et al. Bandage soft contact lenses for ocular graft-versus-dost disease. *Biol Blood Marrow Transplant.* 2015;21(11):2002-2007.
14. Russo PA, Bouchard CS, Galasso JM. Extended-wear silicone hydrogel soft contact lenses in the management of moderate to severe dry eye signs and symptoms secondary to graft-versus-host disease. *Eye Contact Lens.* 2007;33(3):144-147.
15. Schornack MM, Baratz KH, Patel SV, Maguire LJ. Jupiter scleral lenses in the management of chronic graft versus host disease. *Eye Contact Lens.* 2008;34(6):302-305.
16. Theophanous C, Irvine JA, Parker P, Chiu GB. Use of prosthetic replacement of the ocular surface ecosystem scleral lenses in patients with ocular chronic graft-versus-host disease. *Biol Blood Marrow Transplant.* 2015;21(12):2180-2184.
17. Jacobs DS, Rosenthal P. Boston Scleral Lens prosthetic device for treatment of severe dry eye in chronic graft-versus-host disease. *Cornea.* 2007;26(10):1195-1199.
18. DeLoss KS, Le HG, Gire A, Chiu GB, Jacobs DS, Carrasquillo KG. PROSE treatment for Ocular chronic graft-versus-host disease as a clinical network expands. *Eye Contact Lens.* 2016;42(4):262-266.
19. Chiu GB, Theophanous C, Irvine JA. PROSE treatment in atypical ocular graft-versus-host disease. *Optom Vis Sci.* 2016;93(11):1444-1448.
20. Li J, Zhang X, Zheng Q, Zhu Y, Wang H, Ma H, Jhanji V, Chen W. Comparative evaluation of silicone hydrogel contact lenses and autologous serum for management of sjögren syndrome-associated dry eye. *Cornea.* 2015;34(9):1072-1078.
21. Dimit R, Gire A, Pflugfelder SC, Bergmanson JP. Patient ocular conditions and clinical outcomes using a PROSE scleral device. *Cont Lens Anterior Eye.* 2013;36(4):159-163.
22. Romero-Rangel T, Stavrou P, Cotter J, Rosenthal P, Baltatzis S, Foster CS. Gas-permeable scleral contact lens therapy in ocular surface disease. *Am J Ophthalmol.* 2000;130(1):25-32.
23. Pullum K, Buckley R. Therapeutic and ocular surface indications for scleral contact lenses. *Ocul Surf.* 2007;5(1):40-8.
24. Stason WB, Razavi M, Jacobs DS, Shepard DS, Suaya JA, Johns L, Rosenthal P. Clinical benefits of the Boston Ocular Surface Prosthesis. *Am J Ophthalmol.* 2010;149(1):54-61.

25. Lee YK, Lin YC, Tsai SH, Chen WL, Chen YM. Therapeutic outcomes of combined topical autologous serum eye drops with silicone-hydrogel soft contact lenses in the treatment of corneal persistent epithelial defects: A preliminary study. *Cont Lens Anterior Eye.* 2016;39(6):425-430.

26. Schrader S, Wedel T, Moll R, Geerling G. Combination of serum eye drops with hydrogel bandage contact lenses in the treatment of persistent epithelial defects. *Graefes Arch Clin Exp Ophthalmol.* 2006;244(10):1345-1349.

27. Rosenthal P, Cotter JM, Baum J. Treatment of persistent corneal epithelial defect with extended wear of a fluid-ventilated gas-permeable scleral contact lens. *Am J Ophthalmol.* 2000;130(1):33-41.

28. Lim P, Ridges R, Jacobs DS, Rosenthal P. Treatment of persistent corneal epithelial defect with overnight wear of a prosthetic device for the ocular surface. *Am J Ophthalmol.* 2013;156(6):1095-1101.

29. Gumus K, Gire A, Pflugfelder SC. The successful use of Boston ocular surface prosthesis in the treatment of persistent corneal epithelial defect after herpes zoster ophthalmicus. *Cornea.* 2010;29(12):1465-1468.

30. Ling JD, Gire A, Pflugfelder SC. PROSE therapy used to minimize corneal trauma in patients with corneal epithelial defects. *Am J Ophthalmol.* 2013;155(4):615-619.

31. Ciralsky JB, Chapman KO, Rosenblatt MI, Sood P, Fernandez AG, Lee MN, Sippel KC. Treatment of refractory persistent corneal epithelial defects: a standardized approach using continuous wear PROSE therapy. *Ocul Immunol Inflamm.* 2015;23(3):219-224.

CHAPTER 17

Amniotic Membrane for Dry Eye

Elyse J. McGlumphy, MD and Bennie H. Jeng, MD

KEY POINTS

- Amniotic membrane (AM) applied to the ocular surface has been shown to have anti-inflammatory, anti-angiogenic, and anti-scarring properties.
- AM serves as a physical barrier on the ocular surface preventing mechanical eyelid trauma to the epithelium and promoting a protected healing environment.
- AM is commercially available for both in-office (self-retained, sutureless) and procedure room use.

Dry eye syndrome (DES) is one of the most common ocular diagnoses in patients seeking eye care. The incidence of dry eye is higher among females, but both sexes experience an increased incidence with aging. By the 8th to 9th decade of life, conservative estimates suggest approximately 9.8% and 7.7% of women and men, respectively, will experience DES, highlighting the overall significance from a public health perspective.[1] Among the larger studies performed, it has been suggested that in the United States, there may be as many as 5 million individuals over the age of 50 with DES.[2] Using estimates from a 2008 study, the fiscal burden of DES on health care suggest an annual

Mah FS, Rhee MK, eds.
Dry Eye Disease: A Practical Guide (pp 199-208).
© 2019 Taylor & Francis Group.

expense of approximately $3.84 billion from DES alone.[3] The individual economic annual burden has been reported to range from $678 to $1,267 based on the severity of the disease.[4] Over the last decade, the pathogenesis of DES has become better understood, and inflammation has been implicated as a component in several types of dry eye. As such, treatment modalities have been directed specifically at the inflammatory aspects of the disease.

Amniotic Membrane

Amniotic membrane (AM) is a layer of the innermost aspect of the placenta, consisting of an avascular stromal layer with a thick basement membrane. In vivo, AM is pivotal in maintaining the structural integrity of fetal membranes until term, and therefore must prevent inflammation of the secretion of proteolytic proteins to avoid premature rupture of fetal membranes.[5]

Medical Uses

AM use in surgery dates back over 100 years when it was used for dermatologic transplantation.[6] AM was later being utilized in burn care as a wound dressing and had been reported to promote epithelialization, aid with pain relief, and prevent infection.[7] Since then, AM has been studied extensively and has been found to have low immunogenicity, anti-inflammatory, and anti-fibrotic properties all of which support its use as an ideal allograft.

The use of AM in ophthalmology dates back to the 1940s when it was first introduced by de Rötth in conjunctival reconstruction and treatment of persistent corneal defects[8]; however the success rate was reportedly low.[9] Mention of AM use in ophthalmology diminished for many years until 1992 when Dr. Juan Batlle presented at the American Academy of Ophthalmology annual meeting on the ophthalmic uses of AM. Tseng and Kim were pivotal in bringing AM to the forefront in ophthalmology in 1995. Currently, AM is widely used in pterygium excision, for reconstruction of the conjunctival surface, in patients with limbal stem cell deficiencies, and in the treatment of corneal ulcerations as a temporizing or permanent treatment option.[10] It is also frequently used for nonhealing corneal epithelial defects. Most current uses of AM involve some sort of attachment to the ocular surface with adhesive or sutures. There has also been new interest in using a sutureless application of AM for treatment of ocular surface disease.

Preserved AM grafts have been found to express several growth factors including high levels of epithelial growth factor, keratinocyte growth factor, hepatic growth factor, and basic fibroblast growth factor which were higher in grafts containing intact AM epithelium. These growth factors are likely helpful for promoting corneal epithelialization and in corneal wound healing.[11] The anti-proteolytic properties of AM have also been studied and attributed to the expression of tissue inhibitors of metalloproteinases (TIMPS) -1, -2, and -4 which could play a role in preventing proteolytic degradation of tissue.[5] Studies have examined the role of AM's anti-proteolytic properties to determine if these properties translate in grafts and found that corneal proteinase activity was limited and decreased during wound healing in eyes that were patched with AM after chemical injury.[12]

Forms of Amniotic Membrane

Multiple forms of AM have been investigated for use in eye disease. To maximize the biologic benefit of AM in ocular surface disease, it would be most ideal to apply fresh AM, however, this would be logistically and technically impractical due to variability in timing of tissue availability and inadequate time to assure proper screening for communicable diseases. To employ regular use of AM, preservation techniques through cryopreservation or cryodesiccation have been employed to maximize tissue shelf life between harvesting and application. Studies have shown that preserved AM are clinically comparable to fresh AM.[13,14] Cryopreservation of AM is achieved by placing tissue at -80°C for more prolonged storage; AM can be stored for up to 1 month before use at 4°C, easily achieved by most commercially available freezers.[15] Cryodesiccation of AM was introduced as an alternative form of preservation which would allow more flexibility for tissue storage and transport and avoid the need for specialized freezers.[16] AM is sterilized and then subjected to lyophilization or cryodesiccation. There is some concern that cryodesiccation could compromise health of the grafts, but available studies suggest that cryodesiccation of AM is comparable to cryopreservation in maintaining physical, biological, and morphologic characteristics of the tissue.[17] Additional modifications to the cryodesiccation technique using pretreatment of AM with trehalose was shown to be superior in maintaining the morphologic integrity of the tissue and was felt to be structurally comparable to fresh AM—it has also been suggested as a superior alternative to cryopreservation with respect to biocompatibility.[18,19]

Techniques for Application on the Eye

Whether cryopreserved or desiccated, application of AM to the ocular surface can be performed via an inlay technique as a scaffold for epithelialization, the overlay or patch technique as a biologic contact lens, or via a layering technique to fill a large surface defect. The use of AM on the ocular surface is largely employed using fixation techniques to anchor the graft in place using sutures or adhesives. (Figures 17-1A and 17-1B). AM grafts for this use are commercially available and utilized most frequently. Less invasive options of AM application are also available commercially and are a newer technology in the arsenal of treatment. AmbioDisk (Katena Products) is a small dehydrated graft which can be applied directly to the ocular surface and stabilized by placing an overlaying bandage contact lens; one limitation of this product is that it does require fixation via lens or sutures. An entirely sutureless, self-retained, AM graft is also available commercially as PROKERA (Bio-Tissue), initially developed under the name

Figure 17-1. (A) Removal of cryopreserved AM from filter paper backing to treat a nonhealing corneal epithelial defect. (B) AM applied onto eye in preparation for suture fixation in the operating room.

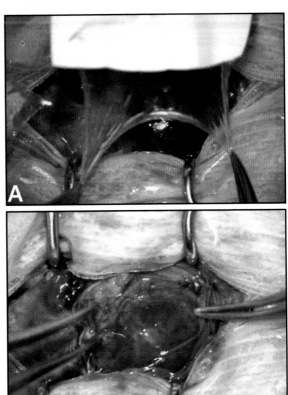

AmnioClip during clinical trials. The polymethyl methacrylate ring system mounts AM and facilitates retention of the AM graft in the eye for up to 1 week, in most patients, before replacement is required, and has shown to have promising effects on corneal surface disease (Table 17-1).[20]

Other Methods of Amniotic Membrane Use

Given the idea that AM harbors important cytokines and growth factors, investigators have sought to determine if AM could be applied in a medium that would maximize the biologic benefits without necessarily worrying about the fixation technique. Creating a homogenate/suspension of AM for use as an eye drop has been suggested to be as effective in healing corneal epithelial damage. In a 2011 study using rabbits, Guo and associates found that AM homogenate was as effective as transplanted AM in promoting corneal healing.[21] Homogenized AM analysis did reveal the presence of growth factors including epidermal growth factor, fibroblast growth factor basic, and hepatocyte growth factor.[22] AM suspension was applied in vitro using human corneal epithelial cultured cells and found to maintain a beneficial effect on corneal epithelial wound healing with significant increases in epithelial migration and proliferation and positive dose response with increased AM concentrations.[23] Morselized AM, in combination with morselized umbilical cord, have in fact been shown to promote rapid epithelialization in patients with refractory corneal epithelial defects.[24] AM is frequently applied to the ocular surface using glue or sutures, but newer sutureless options are available, and there may be a role for use of AM homogenates, as well.

AMNIOTIC MEMBRANE AND DRY EYE SYNDROME

Extending applications of AM use in ocular surface disease to conditions such as dry eye is a novel approach to treatment with promising early outcomes. The application of cryopreserved AM on the ocular surface has been shown to have anti-inflammatory, anti-angiogenic, and anti-scarring properties when transplanted. The anti-inflammatory components of AM could suggest a powerful role for its use in DES given the known role of inflammation in this condition. AM also serves as a physical barrier on the ocular surface preventing mechanical eyelid trauma to the epithelium and thus promoting a protected healing environment.

Despite the theoretical benefits, there is very limited data and research available on the role of AM in treatment of DES. Clinical applications and studies of AM are largely focused on transplantation and/or surgical incorporation of grafts for advanced stages of ocular surface disease; however, groups have started to investigate the role of AM in DES. A recent study by Cheng and colleagues in a group of 15 eyes showed that application of a self-retained cryopreserved AM graft in patients with moderate to severe dry eye for approximately 4.9 days resulted in up to 4 months of symptom improvement with reduction in Ocular Surface Disease Index scores, reduction in use of topical medications, and reduced conjunctival hyperemia.[25] This study, while promising, had a small sample size, and thus was not alone sufficient to support AM use in DES. Other studies have investigated sutureless AM transplantation in patients with severe dry eye due to Stevens-Johnson syndrome and found there was reduction of inflammation and symptomatic relief from dry eye in 14 of 14 treated eyes.[26]

In the future, if data does show a benefit of amniotic membrane transplantation in DES, it may be a plausible new treatment of severe dry eye especially given the advancements in application with a sutureless approach. However, to date, there is not sufficient research or evidence to recommend AM for use in DES, but the limited data available does suggest a promising potential for AM use.

AMNIOTIC MEMBRANE FOR TREATING COMPLICATIONS OF DRY EYE SYNDROME

Although there is limited data for a role for AM in the treatment of DES, AM does have a more established role in treating complications of severe DES. Among indications for AM transplantation, disorders of the cornea represent approximately 41% of cases.[27] The corneal epithelium is an important protective barrier and plays a large role in the stability of the ocular surface. Corneal epithelial defects can develop from dry

TABLE 17-1

CURRENT COMMERCIALLY AVAILABLE AMNIOTIC MEMBRANES AND CHARACTERISTICS

BRAND NAME	MANUFACTURER	PRODUCT VARIATIONS	PROCESSING TECHNIQUE	FIXATION TECHNIQUE	STORAGE METHOD	SHELF LIFE
AmnioGraft	Bio-Tissue	1.5 x 1.0 cm 2.0 x 1.5 cm 2.5 x 2.0 cm 3.5 x 3.5 cm 5.0 x 5.0 cm	Cryopreserved	Suture Adhesive Bandage contact lens	-80°C to -4°C	2 years
PROKERA	Bio-Tissue	Standard Slim Plus	Cryopreserved	Self-retaining	-80°C to -4°C	2 years
AmnioGuard	Bio-Tissue	1.0 x 0.75 cm	Cryopreserved	Suture Adhesive Bandage contact lens	-80°C to -4°C	2 years
Ambio5	Katena Products	1.5 x 2.0 cm 2.0 x 3.0 cm 4.0 x 4.0 cm	Desiccated	Suture Adhesive Bandage contact lens	RT	5 years
Ambio2	Katena Products	1.5 x 2.0 cm 2.0 x 3.0 cm 4.0 x 4.0 cm	Desiccated	Suture Adhesive Bandage contact lens	RT	5 years

Product	Company	Sizes	Processing	Application	Storage	Shelf life
AmbioDisk (device enabling self-retention of Ambio5 or Ambio2)	Katena Products	Ambio2 15 mm disc Ambio5 15 mm disc Ambio2 9 mm disc Ambio2 12 mm disc	Desiccated	Self-retaining	RT	5 years
Aril	Blythe Medical	8 mm disc 10.5 mm disc 15.0 mm disc 1.0 x 2.0 cm ellipse 2.0 x 3.0 cm ellipse	Desiccated Decellularized	Suture Adhesive Bandage contact lens	RT	5 years
BioDOptix	BioD	1.5 x 2.0 cm 2.0 x 3.0 cm 9.0 mm disc 12.0 mm disc 15.0 mm disc	Desiccated	Suture Adhesive Bandage contact lens	RT	5 years
VisiDisc	Skye Biologics	Thin/Thick 10.0 mm disc 12.0 mm disc 15.0 mm disc	Desiccated	Suture Adhesive Bandage contact lens	RT	5 years
OculoMatrix	Skye Biologics	1.0 x 1.0 cm 2.0 x 1.5 cm 2.0 x 2.0 cm 2.0 x 4.0 cm 4.0 x 4.0 cm	Desiccated	Suture Adhesive Bandage contact lens	RT	5 years
AmnioTek-C/AmnioTek	SWISSMED	AmnioTek-C 12 mm disc AmnioTek 3.0 x 3.0 cm	Desiccated	Suture Adhesive Bandage contact lens	RT	3 years

eyes, and if they fail to heal, they can lead to several complications including ulceration, descemetoceles, or even perforation. AM transplantation in patients with persistent corneal epithelial defects, with or without ulceration, serves as an adjunctive basement membrane and thus a scaffold for re-epithelialization.[28]

Similar success with AM has been reported in severe ocular surface disease with nontraumatic corneal perforations and deep ulcers.[29] For deeper ulcerations, a layering technique has been used to fill deeper corneal defects from small perforations, ulcerations, and descemetoceles—with one retrospective study showing 82% rate of closure in 34 eyes treated.[29]

SUMMARY

Most of the current research and studies on AM use in ocular surface disease addresses pathologies on the severe end of the spectrum without an abundance of data on AM use in milder ocular surface disease such as DES. Despite the significant public health burden of DES, topical treatment options remain somewhat limited. The most utilized treatment options are largely limited to supplemental topical lubricants with escalation of therapy for selected patients to topical immunosuppressant/anti-inflammatory medications. Antibiotics with anti-inflammatory profiles including tetracyclines and macrolides have also been used to target the inflammatory component of DES.[30] Topical low dose steroids are also utilized for short-term treatment with good results but also carry a larger side effect profile.[31] Currently, there are 2 FDA approved anti-inflammatory drugs for DES treatment, low dose cyclosporine A 0.05% (Restasis, Allergan), and the more recently approved lifitegrast 5% (Xiidra, Shire). Both drugs target components of the inflammatory cascade with overall effect of T-cell inhibition.[32,33] The frequent and recurrent need for topical therapies does pose a substantial economic burden for patients with DES. As less invasive techniques for AM application surface, application of this therapy will become more plausible for milder ocular surface disease. If substantiated, AM use in DES would represent a novel, non-pharmacologic anti-inflammatory treatment and reduce patient medication burden. Application of this graft by the treating provider may also improve treatment outcomes by diminishing reliance on patient compliance and specifically those with activities of daily living limitations and or impaired cognition. More research is needed to elucidate the role of AM in DES and expound on the breadth of application in the wide spectrum of disease states; however the potential application of this technology could be extraordinary.

REFERENCES

1. Barabino S, Labetoulle M, Rolando M, Messmer EM. Understanding symptoms and quality of life in patients with dry eye syndrome. *Ocul Surf.* 2016;3:365-376.
2. Schaumberg DA, Sullivan DA, Buring JE, Dana MR. Prevalence of dry eye syndrome among US women. *Am J Ophthalmol.* 2003;136:318-326.
3. McDonald M, Patel DA, Keith MS, Snedecor SJ. Economic and humanistic burden of dry eye disease in Europe, North America, and Asia: a systematic literature review. *Ocul Surf.* 2016;2:144-167.

4. Yu J, Asche CV, Fairchild CJ. The economic burden of dry eye diseasein the United States: a decision tree analysis. *Cornea*. 2011;30:379-387.

5. Hao Y, Ma DH, Hwang DG, Kim WS, Zhang F. Identification of antiangiogenic and antiinflammatory proteins in human amniotic membrane. *Cornea*. 2000;19(3):348-352.

6. Davis, S. Skin Transplantation: with a review of 550 cases at the Johns Hopkins hospital. *Johns Hopkins Med J.* 1910;15:307-396.

7. Bose B. Burn wound dressing with human amniotic membrane. *Ann R Coll Surg Engl.* 1979;61(6): 444-447.

8. Tseng SC. Amniotic membrane transplantation for ocular surface reconstruction. *Biosci Rep.* 2001; 21(4):481-489.

9. de Rötth A. Plastic repair of conjunctival defects with fetal membrane. *Arch Ophthalmol.* 1940; 23:522-525.

10. Meller D, Pauklin M, Thomasen H, Westekemper H, Steuhl KP. Amniotic membrane transplantation in the human eye. *Dtsch Arztebl Int.* 2011;108(14):243-248.

11. Koizumi NJ, Inatomi TJ, Sotozono CJ, Fullwood NJ, Quantock AJ, Kinoshita S. Growth factor mRNA and protein in preserved human amniotic membrane. *Curr Eye Res.* 2000; 20(3):173-177.

12. Kim JS, Kim JC, Na BK, Jeong JM, Song CY. Amniotic membrane patching promotes healing and inhibits proteinase activity on wound healing following acute corneal alkali burn. *Exp Eye Res.* 2000; 70(3):329-337.

13. Adds PJ, Hunt CJ, Dart JK. Amniotic membrane grafts, "fresh" or frozen? A clinical and in vitro comparison. *Br J Ophthalmol.* 2001;85(8):905-907.

14. Singh R, GuptaP, Kumar P, Kumar A, Chacharkar MP. Properties of air dried processed amniotic membranes under different storage conditions. *Cell Tissue Banking.* 2003;4(2):95-100.

15. Visuthikosol V, Somna R, Nitiyanant P, Navikarn T. The preparation of lyophylised of fetal membrane for biological dressing. *J Med Assoc Thai.* 1992;75(Suppl 1):52-9.

16. Libera RD, de Melo GB, de Souza Lima A, Haapalainen EF, Cristovam P, Gomes JAP. Assessment of the use of cryopreserved xfreeze-dried amniotic membrane (AM) for reconstruction of ocular surface in rabbit model. *Arq Bras Oftalmol.* 2008;71(5):669-673.

17. Nakamura T, Yoshitani M, Rigby H, Fullwood NJ, Ito W, Inatomi T, Sotozono C, Nakamura T, Shimizu Y, Kinoshita S. Sterilized, freeze-dried amniotic membrane: a useful substrate for ocular surface reconstruction. *Invest Ophthalmol Vis Sci.* 2004;45(1):93-99.

18. Nakamura T, Sekiyama E, Takaoka M, et al., The use of trehalosetreated freeze-dried amniotic membrane for ocular surface reconstruction, *Biomaterials*, 2008;29(27):3729-3737.

19. Allen CL, Clare G, Stewart EA, Branch MJ, McIntosh OD, Dadhwal M, Dua HS, Hopkinson A. Augmented dried versus cryopreserved amniotic membrane as an ocular surface dressing. *PLoS One.* 2013;8(10):e78441.

20. Kotomin I, Valtink M, Hofmann K, Frenzel A, Morawietz H, Werner C, Funk RHW, Engelmann K. Sutureless Fixation of Amniotic Membrane for Therapy of Ocular Surface Disorders. *PLoS One.* 2015;10(5):e0125035.

21. Guo Q, Hao J, Yang Q, Guan L, Ouyang S, Wang J. A comparison of the effectiveness between amniotic membrane homogenate and transplanted amniotic membrane in healing corneal damage in a rabbit model. *Acta Ophthalmol.* 2011;89(4):e315-9.

22. Stachon T, Bischoff M, Seitz B, Huber M, Zawada M, Langenbucher A, Szentmáry N. [Growth Factors and Interleukins in Amniotic Membrane Tissue Homogenate]. [Article in German]. *Klin Monbl Augenheilkd.* 2015;232(7):858-62.

23. Choi JA, Jin HJ, Jung S, et al. Effects of amniotic membrane suspension in human corneal wound healing in vitro. *Mol Vis.* 2009; 15:2230-8.

24. Cheng AMS, Chua L, Casas V, Tseng SCG. Morselized amniotic membrane tissue for refractory corneal epithelial defects in cicatricial ocular surface diseases. *Transl Vis Sci Technol.* 2016;5(3):9.

25. Cheng AM, Zhao D, Chen R, et al. Accelerated restoration of ocular surface health in dry eye disease by self-retained cryopreserved amniotic membrane. *Ocul Surf.* 2016;14(1):56-63.

26. Agrawal A, Pratap VB. Amniotic membrane transplantation (AMT) without the use of sutures/fibrin glue. *Nepal J Ophthalmol.* 2015:7(14):173-177.

27. Tseng SC, Espana EM, Kawakita T, et al. How does amniotic membrane work? *Ocul Surf.* 2004;2(3):177-87.

28. Seitz B. Amniotic membrane transplantation. An indispensable therapy option for persistent corneal epithelial defects. *Ophthalmology.* 2007;104:1075-1079.

29. Solomon A, Meller D, Prabhasawat P, John T, Espana EM, Steuhl KP, Tseng SC. Amniotic membrane grafts for nontraumatic corneal perforations, descemetoceles, and deep ulcers. *Ophthalmology.* 2002;109(4):694-703.

30. Messmer EM. The pathophysiology, diagnosis, and treatment of dry eye disease. *Dtsch Arztebl Int.* 2015;112(5):71-82.

31. Marsh P, Pflugfelder SC. Topical nonpreserved methylprednisolone therapy for keratoconjunctivitis sicca in Sjögren syndrome. *Ophthalmology.* 1999;106(4):811-816.

32. Mah F, Milner M, Yiu S, Donnenfeld E, Conway TM, Hollander DA. PERSIST: Physician's Evaluation of Restasis® Satisfaction in Second Trial of topical cyclosporine ophthalmic emulsion 0.05% for dry eye: a retrospective review. *Clinical Ophthalmology.* 2012;6(1):1971-1976.

33. Holland EJ, Luchs J, Karpecki PM, et al. Lifitegrast for the treatment of dry eye disease: results of a Phase III, randomized, double-masked, placebo-controlled trial (OPUS-3). *Ophthalmology.* 2017;124(1):53-60.

CHAPTER 18

The "Eyelid Facial"
A Review of Meibomian Gland Heat Treatments LipiFlow, MiBo Thermoflo, and Intense Pulsed Light

Morgan R. Godin, MD; Preeya K. Gupta, MD; and Terry Kim, MD

KEY POINTS

◆ Technologies such as thermal pulsation (LipiFlow, TearScience and MiBo Thermoflo, Mibo Medical Group) and intense pulsed light (IPL, DermaMed Solutions) therapy have a role in the treatment of meibomian gland dysfunction (MGD).

◆ The goal temperature to liquefy meibum is 41°C to 43°C.

◆ By ablating eyelid margin telangiectasias, IPL may decrease the inflammatory mediators that are brought to the meibomian glands.

Meibomian gland dysfunction (MGD) is defined as "a chronic diffuse abnormality of the meibomian glands commonly characterized by terminal duct obstruction and/or qualitative/quantitative changes in the glandular secretion."[1] According to conclusions by the recent International Workshop on Meibomian Gland Dysfunction, MGD is the leading cause of evaporative dry eye.[1] Dry eye disease is a multifactorial process that affects millions of people worldwide.[2] Conventional methods for treating MGD and dry eye include warm compresses, eyelid scrubs, artificial tears/gel/ointment, topical

Mah FS, Rhee MK, eds.
Dry Eye Disease: A Practical Guide (pp 209-216).
© 2019 Taylor & Francis Group.

Figure 18-1. LipiFlow Activator eye piece as seen from posterior (A) and anterior (B) views. The eyelid warmer is inserted under the patient's eyelids. The eyecup stays outside the eyelids and inflates to provide manual expression of meibomian glands.[3]

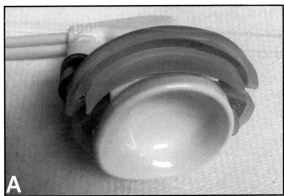

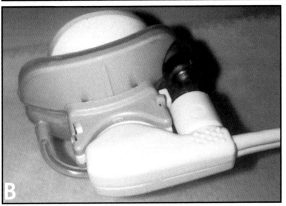

steroids, oral tetracyclines, omega-3 supplementation, environmental modifications, punctal plugs, cyclosporine A 0.5%, lifitegrast 5%, serum tears, etc. However, these treatments are often insufficient. Not only are patients often noncompliant with time-consuming treatment recommendations, but importantly, many of these therapies only address the external ocular surface and do not address the root cause of the disease: deeper obstruction of the meibomian glands. Newer noninvasive treatment device technologies have been developed to provide more effective, consistent, and longer-lasting treatment for MGD. In this chapter, we will discuss thermal pulsation (ie, LipiFlow, MiBo Thermoflo) and intense pulsed light (IPL) therapies.

LipiFlow

LipiFlow is a relatively new in-office treatment designed to relieve meibomian gland obstruction and administer safe and consistent amounts of heat and massage/pressure to the eyelids.

The LipiFlow device consists of a single-use activator eyepiece (one for each eye) and a control system. Each eyepiece contains 2 parts, the eyelid warmer and the eyecup (see Figure 18-1). The eyelid warmer is inserted under the upper and lower eyelids and

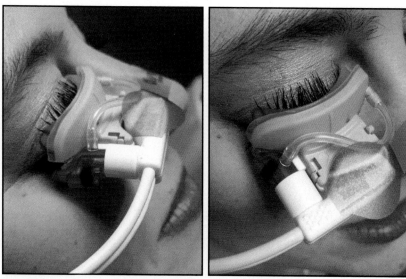

Figure 18-2. LipiFlow eyepieces correctly placed on patient's eyelids.

provides both insulation to protect the globe and heat to the palpebral conjunctival side of the eyelid to liquefy meibum with a goal temperature of 41°C to 43°C. The eyecup sits over the closed eyelids and inflates during treatment in order to compress the eyelids onto the heated eyelid warmer; compression occurs from the base of the glands toward the openings in order to fully express meibum.[3] A critical aspect of the thermal pulsation device is that heat is precisely applied to the posterior aspect of the eyelid, such that it is in close contact with the meibomian glands, allowing for optimal liquefaction of the meibum.

Prior to inserting the eyepieces, topical anesthetic drops should be administered for patient comfort. Once the eyepieces have been appropriately placed, treatment is ready to begin (Figure 18-2). Sessions consist of a 12-minute heat and pressure profile; both eyes are treated simultaneously (Figure 18-3). Patients should be warned that they may experience minor eye irritation after treatment and could notice small subcutaneous hemorrhages at the eyelid margins. In addition, patients should be informed that symptomatic improvement should occur over several weeks following treatment. Follow-up is typically scheduled 2 to 3 months after LipiFlow treatment once the new MGD baseline has been established.

There are multiple controlled studies on the efficacy of LipiFlow. A multicenter trial with 139 MGD patients showed that a single 12-minute LipiFlow treatment significantly improved meibomian gland secretion score, tear break-up time (TBUT), and symptom scores at 2 and 4 weeks post-treatment.[3] Sub-cohorts of 21 and 18 of these patients were evaluated at 9 and 12 months post-treatment, respectively, and found to have persisting improvements in dry eye signs and symptoms.[4-5] Subsequently, 20 patients were studied over the course of 3 years post-LipiFlow and found to have lasting effects with regard to gland secretion (objective) scores and Standard Patient Evaluation of Eye Dryness

Figure 18-3. LipiFlow console showing phase of treatment.

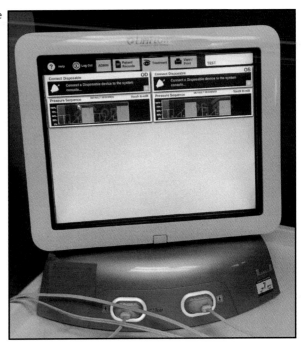

(SPEED) (subjective) scores.[6] Another recent study by a different group of investigators replicated the 1 year results showing that patients had sustained improvement in gland function and reduction in dry eye symptoms.[7] Therefore, LipiFlow's effects typically last up to 1 year (and possibly up to 3 years) before patients feel that another treatment is needed.

MiBo Thermoflo

MiBo Thermoflo combines external heat and pressure to the eyelids to treat MGD. The MiBo Thermoflo device is comprised of a hand piece with 2 pads on its end (Figure 18-4). The technician applies ultrasound gel to these pads and then gently places the pads on the external eyelids (with the eye closed). For maximum efficacy, the eyelash line should be in the space between the pads. Once set up is complete, the warm hand piece is rotated in a circular motion while slowly proceeding along the eyelash line. Light pressure along with heat at 42.5°C help liquefy then express meibomian gland contents. This technology is more operator-dependent than LipiFlow, and care must be taken to maintain the eye pad in even contact with the eyelid skin throughout treatment. Treatment sessions last 24 minutes (12 minutes per eye) with the typical MiBoFlo Thermoflo regimen consisting of 3 to 4 treatments every 2 weeks in order to achieve lasting results.

Overall, there are minimal studies on MiBo Thermoflo in the literature. Recently, one small study of 13 MGD patients who received MiBo Thermoflo treatment to the

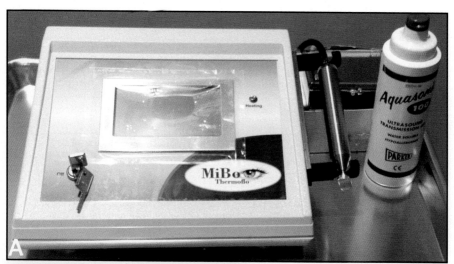

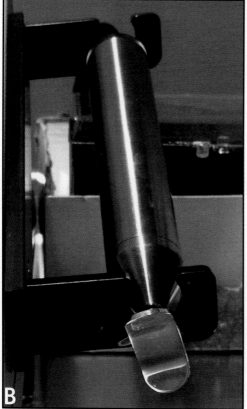

Figure 18-4. (A) MiBo Thermoflo device including console and (B) hand piece with pad on the end.

TABLE 18-1

		FITZPATRICK SCALE		
FITZPATRICK TYPE	**SKIN COLOR**	**TYPICAL HAIR AND EYE COLOR**	**SKIN BEHAVIOR IN SUN**	**OKAY FOR IPL?**
I	Very fair	Blond/red, blue	Always burns, cannot tan	Yes
II	Fair	Blond/light brown, blue/green/hazel	Usually burns, sometimes tans	Yes
III	Medium	Any hair or eye color	Sometimes burns, usually tans	Yes
IV	Olive	Brown, brown	Rarely burns, always tans	Yes
V	Brown	Dark brown, brown	Never burns, always tans	No
VI	Black	Very dark brown, dark brown	Never burns, always tans	No

upper eyelids only showed that all patients reported immediate improvement in symptoms after treatment and had corresponding statistically significant improvement in MGD and blepharitis scores at 4 weeks post-treatment.[8]

INTENSE PULSED LIGHT

The IPL device has historically been used by dermatologists for the treatment of rosacea and facial skin telangiectasias. Light energy is converted to heat and ablates fine vascular structures.[9] The proposed mechanism of action in dry eye is that ablation of eyelid margin telangiectasias decreases inflammatory mediators brought by these vessels to meibomian glands. Furthermore, warming of meibomian glands during the procedure allows for glands to be expressed more easily after the procedure.[10]

Prior to the IPL procedure, eye shields should be applied over the patients' eyelids to protect the underlying eye structures from light energy (Figure 18-5). Providers should also wear appropriate eye goggles for their own eye protection. Initial energy settings are based on patient skin type as determined by the Fitzpatrick scale (settings 1 to 4, mode A to F) and patient tolerance. Of note, only patients with Fitzpatrick skin type IV or lower are eligible for IPL (Table 18-1).[10-11]

The provider should apply ultrasound gel under the lower eyelids including the lateral canthal area and upper cheeks. The upper eyelids should *not* be directly treated because light energy could damage the cornea or other structures including the iris.

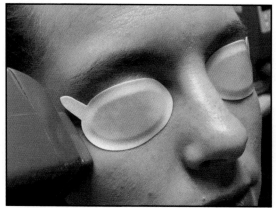

Figure 18-5. IPL treatment application to upper cheek/lateral canthus area with eye shields in place. Note: when actually treating, must apply ultrasound gel to patient's skin.

The IPL hand piece is then used to apply 10 to 15 treatment spots at each of 3 locations: lower eyelid margin, upper cheek (below lower eyelid), and lateral canthal area; 2 passes are made over each of these locations.[12] After the second pass, the eye shields and ultrasound gel are removed. Next, warm compresses are applied to the eyelids followed by topical anesthetic drops and manual expression of meibomian glands with cotton tip applicators. Often, patients are prescribed loteprednol 0.5% twice a day for 2 to 3 days post-procedure. The IPL regimen for dry eye includes an initiation treatment followed by 3 to 6 additional treatments every 4 to 6 weeks, and patients usually find that symptoms improve after their initial series of treatments. Patients get relief from dry eye symptoms typically for several months with a single maintenance treatment every 6 months or more.

Peer-reviewed research has been done on IPL therapy for dry eye. Gupta et al showed that after an average of 4 IPL sessions, there was significant decrease in eyelid margin edema and vascularity, meibum viscosity, and Ocular Surface Disease Index (OSDI) score as well as an increase in oil flow and TBUT.[10] In addition, Craig et al reported a prospective paired-eye study of 28 patients undergoing IPL which showed improvement in lipid layer grade and TBUT in the treated eye but not in the control; furthermore, 86% of participants reported reduced dry eye symptoms in the treated eye.[13] Finally, Toyos et al[12] performed a retrospective study of 91 severe dry eye patients that had IPL monthly until adequate improvement in dry eye syndrome was achieved, based on physician judgment. On average, after 7 treatment visits and 4 maintenance visits over the course of 3 years, 87% of patients had improvement in TBUT, and 93% reported post-treatment satisfaction. Adverse events including redness and swelling were found in 13% of patients with no serious adverse events reported.[12]

SUMMARY

There are several modern noninvasive external treatment technologies designed to improve dry eye disease. While appropriate patient selection is important and cost may be prohibitive for some patients, these treatments should be discussed with all patients who suffer from MGD as earlier intervention tends to yield better results and can help to hold off progressive gland atrophy and inflammation. Numerous studies in the literature on LipiFlow and IPL therapies show improvement in both signs and symptoms of dry eye disease for months to years following treatment. These procedures also all appear to be safe with minimal adverse reactions.

REFERENCES

1. Nichols KK, Foulks GN, Bron AJ et al. The international workshop on meibomian gland dysfunction: Executive summary. *Invest Ophthalmol Vis Sci.* 2011;52:1922-1929.
2. Lemp MA, Baudouin C, Baum J et al. The definition and classification of dry eye disease: reports of the Definition and Classification Subcommittee of the International Dry Eye Workshop. *Ocul Surf.* 2007;5(2):75-92.
3. Lane SS, DuBiner HB, Epstein RJ et al. A new system, the Lipiflow, for the treatment of meibomian gland dysfunction. *Cornea.* 2012;31(4):396-404.
4. Greiner JV. A singly Lipiflow® thermal pulsation system treatment improves meibomian gland function and reduces dry eye symptoms for 9 months. *Curr Eye Res.* 2012;37(4):272-278.
5. Greiner JV. Long-term (12 month) improvement in meibomian gland function and reduced dry eye symptoms with a single thermal pulsation treatment. *Clin Ecp Ophthalmol.* 2013;41(6):524-530.
6. Greiner JV. Long-term (3 year) effects of a single thermal pulsation system treatment on meibomian gland function and dry eye symptoms. *Eye Contact Lens.* 2016;42(2):99-107.
7. Blackie CA, Coleman CA, Holland EJ. The sustained effect (12 months) of a single-dose vectored thermal pulsation procedure for meibomian gland dysfunction and evaporative dry eye. *Clin Ophthalmol.* 2016;10:1385-1396.
8. Connor, CG, Narayanan S, Miller WL. The efficacy of MiBoThermoflo in treatment of meibomian gland dysfunction. University of the Incarnate Word Web site. http://www.uiw.edu/optometry/documents/arvoabstracts.pdf. Published May 5, 2016.
9. Kassir R, Kolluru A, Kassir M. Intense pulsed light for the treatment of rosacea and telangiectasias. *J Cosmet Laser Ther.* 2011;13:216-222.
10. Gupta PK, Vora GK, Matossian C, Kim M, Stinnett S. Outcome of intense pulsed light therapy for treatment of evaporative dry eye disease. *Can J Ophthalmol.* 2016;51(4):249-253.
11. Vora GK, Gupta PK. Intense pulsed light therapy for the treatment of evaporative dry eye disease. *Curr Opin Ophthalmol.* 2015;26:314-318.
12. Toyos R, McGill W, Brisoce D. Intense pulsed light treatment for dry eye disease due to meibomian gland dysfunction; a 3 year retrospective study. *Photomed Laser Surg.* 2015;33(1):41-46.
13. Craig JP, Chen YH, Turnbull PRK. Prospective trial of intense pulsed light for the treatment of meibomian gland dysfunction. *Invest Ophthalmol Vis Sci.* 2015;56(3):1965-1970.

CHAPTER 19

Acupuncture for Dry Eye
The Role of Integrative Medicine as an Adjunctive Treatment

Siwei Zhou, MD and Deepinder K. Dhaliwal, MD, LAc

KEY POINTS

- Acupuncture involves the insertion of thin needles into the skin at specific points called acupoints.
- The mechanism of acupuncture may be centered around altering molecular pathways to reduce inflammation and to decrease the sensation of pain.
- Despite the small sample size of studies, there is evidence that acupuncture may improve patient discomfort, corneal staining, and tear break-up time (TBUT).

Acupuncture is thought to have originated over 3000 years ago in China.[1] The foundations of acupuncture were laid out in the classic Chinese texts "Huangdi Neijing" (Inner Classic of Huangdi) and "The Great Compendium of Acupuncture and Moxibustion" written during the Ming dynasty (1368 to 1644).[2] Today, acupuncture is used to treat a variety of disease states, including depression, functional dyspepsia, infertility, and pain disorders such as migraine and low back pain. Complementary

Mah FS, Rhee MK, eds.
Dry Eye Disease: A Practical Guide (pp 217-225).
© 2019 Taylor & Francis Group.

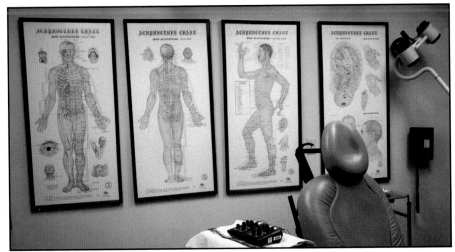

Figure 19-1. Acupoint/meridian maps as displayed at the Center for Integrative Eye Care at the University of Pittsburgh Medical Center.

alternative medicine and acupuncture have also been increasingly popular in the treatment of ocular disorders such as glaucoma[3] and inflammatory eye disease such as dry eye.[4]

WHAT IS ACUPUNCTURE

Acupuncture involves the insertion of thin needles into the skin at specific points called acupoints. There are hundreds of defined acupoints based on the 14 meridians throughout the body[5] (Figure 19-1). It has been proposed that acupoints have a higher density of nerve endings, microvessels, higher concentration of mast cells, and a close relationship to connective tissue planes. Studies have also shown that skin electrical resistance is lower at acupoints in healthy individuals.[5]

Acupuncture needles range from 0.12 to 0.35 mm in thickness and 13 mm to 125 mm in length. There are semipermanent ear needles used in auricular therapy (Figure 19-2). In a typical acupuncture session, needles are placed in a set of acupoints selected for a particular therapeutic goal. Each session is typically 15 to 45 minutes long. The needles may be manipulated by the acupuncturist in a method called "de qi" which involves rotating or twisting the needle up and down.[5] Electrodes may also be connected to the needles to electrically stimulate the acupoints and enhance therapy (Figure 19-3).

MECHANISMS OF ACUPUNCTURE

Several mechanisms of action of acupuncture have been proposed. Acupuncture has been found to decrease proinflammatory cytokines, thereby having an anti-inflammatory

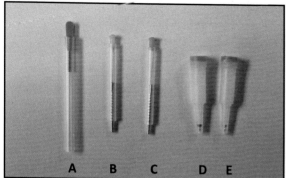

Figure 19-2. Examples of types of acupuncture needles. (A) Seirin L-Type, No. 3, 0.20 x 30 mm. (B) AcuGlide, MT1-2215, 0.22 x 12 mm. (C) AcuGlide, MT1-2015, 0.20 x 15 mm. (D) ASP classic semi permanent acupuncture needles. (E) ASP gold semi permanent acupuncture needles.

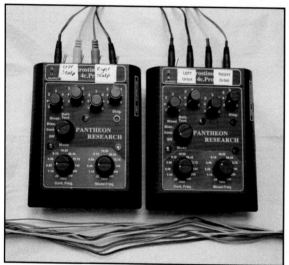

Figure 19-3. Electrodes used in acupuncture therapy.

effect with implications for chronic inflammatory conditions such as inflammatory bowel disease, dry eye, rheumatoid arthritis, and depression.[6-8] Furthermore, acupuncture has been found to increase blood flow to organs,[9] reduce the sensation of pain,[10,11] and modulate the sympathetic system in mechanisms similar to muscle contraction in prolonged exercise.[12] Electrical stimulation of tissue has been found to enhance wound healing by increasing fibroblastic proliferation, inducing cell migration, having antibacterial properties, and increasing revascularization.[13]

A series of studies have analyzed protein expression in blood, urine, and saliva before and after stimulation of the Zusanli (ST-36) point—a point commonly used to treat a wide range of gastrointestinal disorders. The authors concluded that stimulation of the acupoint led to activation of different metabolic pathways.[14-16] The effects of acupuncture have been further validated through neuroimaging studies. Dhond et al reported functional MRI studies in humans which showed immediate effects of prolonged acupuncture stimulation in the limbic and basal forebrain areas related to somatosensory and affective functions known to be involved in pain processing.[17] Harris et al documented that positron-emission tomography has shown acupuncture to increase μ-opioid-binding potential for several days in some of the same brain areas, while also showing distinct changes in limbic structures between true and sham acupuncture.[18]

EVIDENCE FOR ACUPUNCTURE FOR DRY EYE

Several studies have shown benefits of acupuncture in the treatment of dry eye. An observational study of 50 patients by Jeon et al showed that acupuncture significantly improves dry eye symptom scores, Ocular Surface Disease Index (OSDI) scores, and Schirmer test scores, but not tear break-up time (TBUT).[19]

On a molecular level, Qiu et al showed differences in tear protein expression and lacrimal gland function after acupuncture in the animal model.[20] Furthermore, Nepp et al measured corneal tear film in human subjects receiving acupuncture and found an increase in precorneal tear film temperature in subjects receiving acupuncture, as well as statistically significant increases in TBUT and lipid layer thickness, but not in Schirmer II test scores.[21]

Randomized controlled trials have reported acupuncture therapy to show statistically significant improvements on parameters of dry eye compared with artificial tears, but the effect can be delayed.[15,22-26] Gong et al showed that there were significant differences in the acupuncture group compared to the artificial tears control group in symptoms, TBUT, and Schirmer test scores at 3 weeks post-treatment, but not immediately post-treatment.[24] Furthermore, Kim et al[25] showed no improvements in the acupuncture vs artificial tear groups immediately after treatment, but significant improvement in OSDI and visual analog scale (VAS [for self-assessment of ocular discomfort]) in the acupuncture group 8 weeks after the end of acupuncture treatment.

Lin et al randomized 96 patients to receive acupuncture therapy or artificial tears and categorized the patient as having Sjögren syndrome dry eye (SSDE), non-Sjögren syndrome dry eye (non-SSDE) and lipid tear deficiency (LTD).[22] Fourier-domain optical coherence tomography (FD-OCT) was used to measure tear film parameters such as tear meniscus height (TMH), tear meniscus depth (TMD) and tear meniscus area (TMA). The study found that FD-OCT tear film parameters as well as OSDI, TBUT and Schirmer I test scores were significantly improved in the non-SSDE and LTD acupuncture groups compared to the artificial tear control groups, but not in the SSDE acupuncture group. The results suggest that acupuncture therapy may not be equally effective for different types of dry eye and may be of limited value for patients with primary Sjögren syndrome.

A meta-analysis by Tang et al performed on data from 7 randomized controlled trials comparing acupuncture with artificial tears replacement found that acupuncture therapy improved TBUT, Schirmer I test scores, corneal fluorescein staining (CFS), and VAS compared with artificial tears.[27]

Overall, it has been difficult to draw definitive conclusions regarding the efficacy of acupuncture due to the low total number of randomized controlled trials, the small sample sizes of the studies, and lack of true negative controls. Very few trials have been conducted using sham acupuncture as a negative control. Shin et al conducted a randomized placebo-controlled trial with 49 patients and found no significant difference in OSDI, VAS, TBUT, or Schirmer I test scores between the 2 groups.[28] In fact, Lund et al argues that sham acupuncture is not acceptable as placebo controls because even the superficial, minimal sham acupuncture procedures can lead to physiologic change beyond that of a placebo effect.[29,30]

SAFETY OF ACUPUNCTURE

Acupuncture is generally a favorable adjuvant treatment given its safety profile and low incidence of adverse effects. A majority of the adverse effects are mild and transient, including needling pain, bleeding, or bruising at the site of the needle. The incidence of these minor adverse effects was reported in 6.7% of cases in a large prospective study by White et al.[31] Several serious adverse effects that have been associated with acupuncture occurred in the abdominal and thoracic regions, including trauma to internal organs such as pneumothorax or cardiac tamponade, and infections such as hepatitis C or HIV.[2] An early survey by Ernst et al found that serious side effects such as cardiac tamponade, pneumothorax, endocarditis, hepatitis, and spinal lesions are nearly 3 times more common in nonmedically trained acupuncturists than in medically trained acupuncturists.[32] One of the largest prospective observational studies by Witt et al found that of nearly 230,000 patients receiving acupuncture, 8.6% of patients reported experiencing at least 1 adverse effect and 2.2% reported 1 which required treatment.[33] The most common of these adverse effects were bleeding or hematoma (58% of all adverse effects). Overall, acupuncture has been shown to be a relatively safe therapy when performed by physicians, but the potential for adverse effects should be discussed with patients considering acupuncture.

EXAMPLE OF ACUPUNCTURE FOR DRY EYE PROTOCOL

Acupuncture protocols for the treatment of dry eye vary greatly among practitioners. Reported studies have conducted anywhere from 9 to 30 sessions over 10 days to 2 months, each session lasting 20 to 30 minutes and involving 8 to 24 acupoints with or without "de qi."[27,34]

In a recent and currently unpublished study conducted at the Center for Integrative Eye Care at the University of Pittsburgh Medical Center by Dhaliwal et al,[35] 49 patients completed a prospective, randomized, double-blinded sham acupuncture controlled study using the Niemtzow protocol.[36,37] Sterile, disposable, stainless steel acupuncture needles with individual guide tubes were placed for 45 minutes without electrical or manual stimulation. For true acupuncture treatment, a total of 12 needles were placed bilaterally on the ears (at acupuncture points Salivary Gland-2, Point Zero, and Shen Men) and bilaterally on the index fingers (Large Intestine-1 [LI-1], and Large Intestine-2 [LI-2], and between LI-1 and LI-2) (Figure 19-4). For sham acupuncture treatment, 4

Figure 19-4. True acupuncture therapy used by Dhaliwal et al.[35] (A) Auricular points Salivary Gland-2, Point Zero, and Shen Men. (B) Index finger points Large Intestine-1 (LI-1), and Large Intestine-2 (LI-2), and between LI-1 and LI-2).

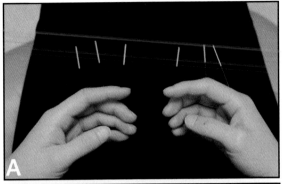

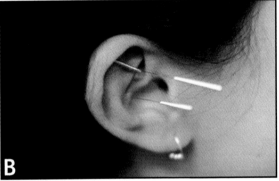

needles were placed bilaterally in a 1-cm circle situated on the left and right upper shoulder areas outside of any known acupuncture points or meridians (Figure 19-5). Each group received 1 acupuncture treatment on 2 consecutive days for a total of 2 treatment sessions per participant. Treatment outcomes were assessed by the OSDI questionnaire, ocular surface staining, tear flow, TBUT, and a general questionnaire.

OSDI scores were found to improve in both treatment and control groups at 1 week, and there was a significant improvement in the OSDI in the treatment group vs the sham group at 6 months ($P=0.04$). There were no significant differences in TBUT, tear flow, and ocular surface grading between the acupuncture and the control groups.

Overall, although there was no difference in the objective measures of dry eye, patients were symptomatically improved for at least 6 months after 2 sessions of acupuncture. Much of the treatment of dry eye is focused on management of symptoms, and therefore, a subjective improvement in eye discomfort in dry eye has a significant impact on decreasing the societal burden of dry eye.

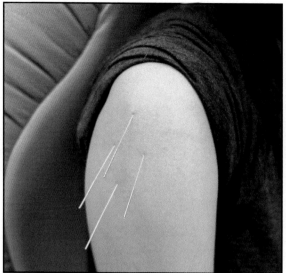

Figure 19-5. Sham Acupuncture Therapy used by Dhaliwal et al.[35] Four needles placed bilaterally in a 1 cm circle situated on the left and right upper shoulder areas outside of any known acupuncture points or meridians.

SUMMARY

The mechanisms of acupuncture are still widely unknown but may be centered around altering molecular pathways to reduce inflammation and to decrease the sensation of pain. There are limitations in our understanding of the therapy due to lack of appropriate power of studies and lack of a true negative control for acupuncture. Overall, acupuncture therapy is a relatively safe option for patients who suffer from the symptoms of dry eye and are willing to try complementary medicine as a supplement to their current dry eye therapy.

REFERENCES

1. White A, Ernst E. A brief history of acupuncture. *Rheumatology.* 2004;43(5):662-663.
2. Ernst E. Acupuncture - a critical analysis. *J Intern Med.* 2006;259(2):125-137.
3. Rhee DJ, Spaeth GL, Myers JS, et al. Prevalence of the use of complementary and alternative medicine for glaucoma. *Ophthalmology.* 2002;109:438-443.
4. Smith JR, Spurrier NJ, Martin JT, Rosenbaum JT. Prevalent use of complementary and alternative medicine by patients with inflammatory eye disease. *Ocul Immunol Inflamm.* 2004;12(3):203-214.
5. Li F, He T, Xu Q, et al. What is the acupoint? A preliminary review of acupoints. *Pain Med.* 2015;16(10):1905-1915.
6. Lu J, Shao R-H, Hu L, Tu Y, Guo J-Y. Potential antiinflammatory effects of acupuncture in a chronic stress model of depression in rats. *Neurosci Lett.* 2016;618:31-38.
7. Oke SL, Tracey KJ. The inflammatory reflex and the role of complenetary and alternative medical therapies. *Ann N Y Acad Sci.* 2009;1172:172-180.
8. Kavoussi B, Ross BE. The neuroimmune basis of anti-inflammatory acupuncture. *Integr Cancer Ther.* 2007;6(3):251-257.

9. Uchida S, Hotta H. Acupuncture affects regional blood flow in various organs. *Evid Based Complement Alternat Med.* 2008;5(2):145-151.
10. Bäcker M, Grossman P, Schneider J, et al. Acupuncture in migraine: investigation of autonomic effects. *Clin J Pain.* 2008;24(2):106-115.
11. Nepp J, Jandrasits K, Schauersberger J, et al. Is acupuncture a useful tool for pain-treatment in ophthalmology? *Acupunct Electrother Res.* 2002;27(3-4):171-182.
12. Andersson S, Lundeberg T. Acupuncture - from empiricism to science: functional background to acupuncture effects in pain and disease. *Med Hypotheses.* 1995;45(3):271-281.
13. Kloth LC. Electrical stimulation for wound healing: a review of evidence from in vitro studies, animal experiments, and clinical trials. *Int J Low Extrem Wounds.* 2005;4(1):23-44.
14. Yan G, Zhang A, Sun H, et al. Dissection of biological property of chinese acupuncture point zusanli based on long-term treatment via modulating multiple metabolic pathways. *Evid Based Complement Alternat Med.* 2013;2013:429703.
15. Zhang Y, Yang W. Effects of acupuncture and moxibustion on tear-film of the patients with xerophthalmia. *J Tradit Chin Med.* 2007;27(4):258-260.
16. Zhang Y, Zhang A, Yan G, et al. High-throughput metabolomic approach revealed the acupuncture exerting intervention effects by perturbed signatures and pathways. *Mol Biosyst.* 2014;10(1):65-73.
17. Dhond RP, Kettner N, Napadow V. Neuroimaging acupuncture effects in the human brain. *J Altern Complement Med.* 2007;13(6):603-616.
18. Harris RE, Zubieta JK, Scott DJ, Napadow V, Gracely RH, Clauw DJ. Traditional Chinese acupuncture and placebo (sham) acupuncture are differentiated by their effects on mu-opioid receptors (MORs). *Neuroimage.* 2009;47(3):1077-1085.
19. Jeon J-H, Shin M-S, Lee MS, et al. Acupuncture reduces symptoms of dry eye syndrome: a preliminary observational study. *J Altern Complement Med.* 2010;16(12):1291-1294.
20. Qiu X, Gong L, Sun X, Guo J, Chodara AM. Efficacy of acupuncture and identification of tear protein expression changes using iTRAQ quantitative proteomics in rabbits. *Curr Eye Res.* 2011;36(10):886-894.
21. Nepp J, Tsubota K, Goto E, et al. The effect of acupuncture on the temperature of the ocular surface in conjunctivitis sicca measured by non-contact thermography: preliminary results. *Adv Exp Med Biol.* 2AD;506:723-726.
22. Lin T, Gong L, Liu X, Ma X. Fourier-domain optical coherence tomography for monitoring the lower tear meniscus in dry eye after acupuncture treatment. *Evid Based Complement Alternat Med.* 2015;2015:492150.
23. Grönlund MA, Stenevi U, Lundeberg T. Acupuncture treatment in patients with keratoconjunctivitis sicca: a pilot study. *Acta Ophthalmol Scand.* 2004;82:283-290.
24. Gong L, Sun X, Chapin WJ. Clinical curative effect of acupuncture therapy on xerophthalmia. *Am J Chin Med.* 2010;38(4):651-659.
25. Kim TH, Kang JW, Kim KH, et al. Acupuncture for the treatment of dry eye: A multicenter randomised controlled trial with active comparison intervention (artificial teardrops). *PLoS One.* 2012;7(5):1-9.
26. Nepp J, Wedrich A, Akramian J, et al. Dry eye treatment with acupuncture. A prospective, randomized, double-masked study. *Adv Exp Med Biol.* 1998;438:1011-1016.
27. Yang L, Yang Z, Yu H, Song H. Acupuncture therapy is more effective than artificial tears for dry eye syndrome: Evidence based on a meta-analysis. *Evid Based Complement Alternat Med.* 2015;2015:1438585.
28. Shin MS, Kim JI, Lee MS, et al. Acupuncture for treating dry eye: A randomized placebo-controlled trial. *Acta Ophthalmol.* 2010;88(8):328-333.
29. Lund I, Näslund J, Lundeberg T. Minimal acupuncture is not a valid placebo control in randomised controlled trials of acupuncture: A physiologist's perspective. *Dtsch Zeitschrift fur Akupunkt.* 2009;52(2):55-56.
30. Lund I, Lundeberg T. Are minimal, superficial or sham acupuncture procedures acceptable as inert placebo controls? *Acupunct Med.* 2006;24(1):13-15.
31. White A, Hayhoe S, Hart A, Ernst E. Adverse events following acupuncture: prospective survey of 32000 consultations with doctors and physiotherapists. *Bristish Med J.* 2001;323(7311):485-486.

32. Ernst E, White A. Life-threatening adverse reactions after acupuncture? A systematic review. *Pain.* 1997;71(2):123-126.

33. Witt CM, Pach D, Brinkhaus B, et al. Safety of acupuncture: Results of a prospective observational study with 229,230 patients and introduction of a medical information and consent form. *Forsch Komplementarmed.* 2009;16(2):91-97.

34. Lee MS, Shin BC, Choi TY, Ernst E. Acupuncture for treating dry eye: A systematic review. *Acta Ophthalmol.* 2011;89(2):101-106.

35. Dhaliwal DK, Zhou S, Samudre SS, Lo NJ, Rhee MK. Acupuncture for dry eye: current perspectives. A double-blinded randomized control trial and review of the literature. In press.

36. Niemtzow RC, C MB, P PY, A JP. Acupuncture technique for pilocarpine-resistant xerostomia following radiotherapy for head and neck malignancies. *Med Acupunct.* 2000;12:42-43.

37. Johnstone PAS, Peng YP, May BC, Inouye WS, Niemtzow RC. Acupuncture for pilocarpine-resistant xerostomia following radiotherapy for head and neck malignancies. *Int J Radiat Oncol Biol Phys.* 2001;50(2):353-357.

Financial Disclosures

Dr. Guillermo Amescua has no financial or proprietary interest in the materials presented herein.

Dr. Alex Barsam has not disclosed any relevant financial relationships.

Dr. Ashley R. Brissette is a consultant for Carl Zeiss Meditec, Johnson & Johnson Vision, and conducts research partially funded by Shire.

Dr. Frank X. Cao has no financial or proprietary interest in the materials presented herein.

Dr. Lorenzo J. Cervantes has no financial or proprietary interest in the materials presented herein.

Dr. Audrey A. Chan has no financial or proprietary interest in the materials presented herein.

Dr. Deepinder K. Dhaliwal is a consultant for Bausch + Lomb, a member of the medical advisory board for NovaBay Pharmaceuticals, a speaker for Staar, a researcher for Imprimis for which she receives grants, and AMO Trainer for VISX and Intralase lasers.

Dr. Katherine Duncan has no financial or proprietary interest in the materials presented herein.

Dr. Marjan Farid is a consultant for Allergan, Shire, Johnson & Johnson Vision, Kala Pharmaceuticals, Bio-Tissue, and CorneaGen.

Dr. Anat Galor has no financial or proprietary interest in the materials presented herein.

Dr. Morgan R. Godin has no financial or proprietary interest in the materials presented herein.

Dr. Preeya K. Gupta is a consultant for Johnson & Johnson.

Dr. Albert S. Hazan has no financial or proprietary interest in the materials presented herein.

Dr. Kourtney Houser has no financial or proprietary interest in the materials presented herein.

Dr. Deborah S. Jacobs has no financial or proprietary interest in the materials presented herein.

Dr. Emily J. Jacobs has no financial or proprietary interest in the materials presented herein.

Dr. Bennie H. Jeng has no financial or proprietary interest in the materials presented herein.

Dr. Stephen C. Kaufman has no financial or proprietary interest in the materials presented herein.

Dr. Michelle J. Kim has no financial or proprietary interest in the materials presented herein.

Dr. Terry Kim is a consultant to Aerie Pharmaceuticals, Alcon, Allergan, Avedro, Avellino Labs, Bausch + Lomb, Blephex, Co-Da/Ocunexus Therapeutics, Kala Pharmaceuticals, NovaBay Pharmaceuticals, Ocular Therapeutix, Omeros, PowerVision, Presbyopia Therapies, Shire, SightLife Surgical, Silk Technologies, Simple Contacts, TearLab, TearScience.

Dr. Francis S. Mah is a consultant for Aerie, Alcon, Allergan, Avedro, Avellino Group, Bausch + Lomb, BlephEx, EyePoint Pharmaceuticals, Eyevance Pharmaceuticals, iView, Johnson & Johnson, Kala Pharmaceuticals, Mallinckrodt Pharmaceuticals, Ocular Science, Ocular Therapeutix, Oculonexus, Okogen, Omeros, PMN, PolyActiva, RxSight, Shire, Sun, Sydnexis, TearLab, and TearScience.

Dr. Elyse J. McGlumphy has no financial or proprietary interest in the materials presented herein.

Dr. Sotiria Palioura has no financial or proprietary interest in the materials presented herein.

Dr. Victor L. Perez has not disclosed any relevant financial relationships.

Dr. Stephen C. Pflugfelder is a consultant for Allergan and Senju.

Dr. Nataliya Pokeza has no financial or proprietary interest in the materials presented herein.

Dr. Michelle K. Rhee has no financial or proprietary interest in the materials presented herein.

Dr. Allison Rizzuti has no financial or proprietary interest in the materials presented herein.

Dr. Kelsey Roelofs has no financial or proprietary interest in the materials presented herein.

Dr. Bryan Roth has no financial or proprietary interest in the materials presented herein.

Dr. John Sheppard is a consultant for Alcon, Allergan, Novartis, Bausch + Lomb, Aldeyra Therapeutics, Topivert, Noveome Biotheraputics, Son Pharma, Bruder Healthcare, Tracey Technologies, Hovione, EyePoint, Shire, Doctors Allergy Formula, 1-800-Doctors, Tissue Tech, Mallinckrodt Pharmaceuticals, and Santen Pharmaceutical.

Dr. Patricia B. Sierra has no financial or proprietary interest in the materials presented herein.

Dr. Christopher E. Starr is a consultant for Allergan, Shire, Bausch + Lomb, TearLab, RPS, Sun, Refocus, GlassesOff, Kala Pharmaceuticals, Bruder, Quidel, and Blephex.

Dr. Christos Theophanous has no financial or proprietary interest in the materials presented herein.

Dr. Danielle Trief has no financial or proprietary interest in the materials presented herein.

Dr. Felipe A. Valenzuela has not disclosed any relevant financial relationships.

Dr. Nandini Venkateswaran has no financial or proprietary interest in the materials presented herein.

Dr. Elizabeth Viriya has no financial or proprietary interest in the materials presented herein.

Dr. Priscilla Q. Vu has no financial or proprietary interest in the materials presented herein.

Dr. Walt Whitley is a consultant for Alcon, Allergan, Bausch + Lomb, Bio-Tissue, Beaver-Visitec, Johnson & Johnson Vision, OCuSOFT, Shire, Sun, TearCare, and TearLab.

Dr. Elizabeth Yeu has not disclosed any relevant financial relationships.

Dr. Jenny Y. Yu has no financial or proprietary interest in the materials presented herein.

Dr. Siwei Zhou has not disclosed any relevant financial relationships.

Index

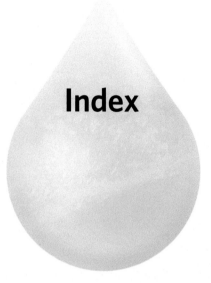

Printed in the United States
by Baker & Taylor Publisher Services